PRETTY SICK

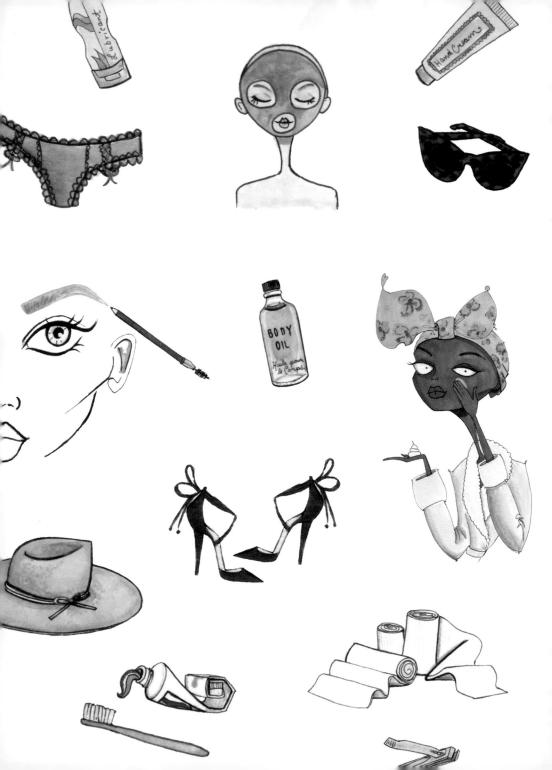

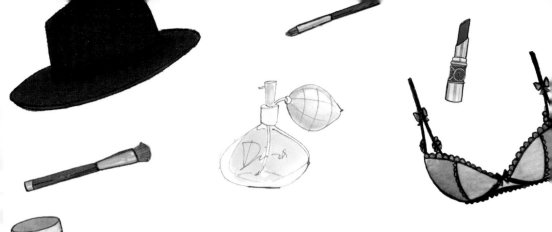

PRETTY SICK

THE BEAUTY GUIDE
for Women with Cancer

Caitlin M. Kiernan

Illustrations by Jamie Lee Reardin

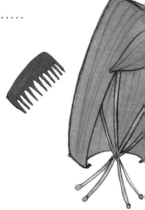

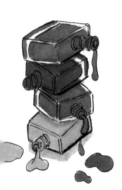

piatkus

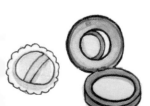

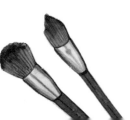

PIATKUS

The information herein is not intended to replace the services of trained health professionals.

You are advised to consult with your health care professional with regard to matters relating to your health, and in particular regarding matters that may require diagnosis or medical attention. The author and publisher disclaim any liability directly or indirectly from the use of the material in this book by any person.

The information provided in this book is based on sources that the author believes to be reliable and the author has attempted to verify its accuracy. All such information regarding individual products and companies is current as of September 2017.

First published in the United States in 2017 by Hachette Book Group, Inc
First published in Great Britain in 2017 by Piatkus

Copyright © 2017 Caitlin M. Kiernan
Illustrations by Jamie Lee Reardin

10 9 8 7 6 5 4 3 2 1

The moral right of the author has been asserted.

Most names have been changed to protect places and people's privacy.

The author has made every effort to ensure the accuracy of the information within this book was correct at time of publication. The author does not assume and hereby disclaim any liability to any party for any loss, damage, or disruption caused by errors or omissions, whether such errors or omissions result from accident, negligence, or any other cause.

A CIP catalogue record for this book is available from the British Library.

Trade Paperback ISBN: 978-0-349-41727-1

Printed and bound in Italy by L.E.G.O. SpA

Papers used by Piatkus are from well-managed forests and other responsible sources.

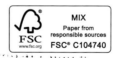

Piatkus
An imprint of
Little, Brown Book Group
Carmelite House
50 Victoria Embankment
London EC4Y 0DZ

An Hachette UK Company
www.hachette.co.uk

www.improvementzone.co.uk

For my grandmother, best friend, and unwavering supporter,

Kathleen "Kay" Kiernan.

I miss you every second of every day.

CONTENTS

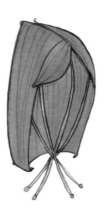

INTRODUCTION

It was gearing up to be one of the biggest events *Life & Style Weekly* magazine had ever held. The Kardashian Klan had RSVP'd. So had all of Bravo's Real Housewives, including NeNe Leakes, Countess Luann de Lesseps, and Ramona Singer. And the fashion world's top stylists—including my friend Robert Verdi—were working the red carpet before it had even been rolled out. The Style Awards party was held to celebrate the magazine's fall fashion issue that was dedicated to Hollywood's most influential trendsetters. Held on the rooftop of the Dream Hotel, the party coincided with New York Fashion Week and was one of the most buzzed about events of the season. *E! News* was there, so was *Entertainment Tonight*, the *New York Post*, the *Daily News*—and a slew of other news organizations. It was set to be one of those magical New York nights.

As the magazine's beauty director, I was responsible for writing and assigning all the beauty coverage in the magazine. It was also part of my job to report on the latest beauty trends, test new products on the market, and to interview celebrities, their glam squads, and the leading experts in the industry. Because of that, I had a hand in nominating and selecting the celebrities and influencers that were going to be featured in our special style issue. And when it came to the party, I helped get these influencers to attend. Not such an easy feat. But collectively, we pulled it off and the night had arrived without any major hitches.

Getting ready for the event was another story. By the night of the party, I was smack-dab in the middle of treatment for breast cancer. I had been diagnosed in July and by September I had already had several surgeries and two rounds of chemotherapy. While getting ready for a dressy event would normally take about an hour, now it took almost three. Chemo made my skin break out in hives and it required time and skills to hide them. Thankfully, I had years of beauty reporting under my belt so I knew how to apply foundation and concealer like a pro. My hair was another matter. I tried, several times, to curl it into sexy, beachy waves. But ever since I started losing clumps at a time, it tended to look limp and lifeless no matter what I did to it. After several frustrating attempts at styling, and close to tears, I pulled it up into a sleek topknot. I finished with a swipe of almost neon orange lipstick. I figured the bold shade, which was totally on trend, would help distract from any obvious signs of my sickness.

Once the doors opened, the room filled with the who's who of the fashion and beauty world. I sipped on a drink and started to work the room. I talked with Khloé Kardashian and Lamar Odom, and neither seemed to notice that I was in the middle of a major health crisis. Khloé complimented my lipstick and my Jimmy Choo heels while we talked about her visiting Lamar's children in Brooklyn. Melissa Gorga and Cindy Barshop, two of Bravo's Real Housewives, grabbed me for an impromptu picture in the photo booth that was rented for the event. After, as we looked at the ten-plus pictures we took, Melissa commented on my glowing skin and asked who my facialist was. My answer: "I don't have one."

It was in that moment that I realized that *nobody* at the party— minus a few of my colleagues—knew I had cancer. I was standing among Hollywood's elite makeup artists, hairstylists, fashion stylists, talent scouts, agents, and celebrities—people who are known for their looks or whose jobs it is to create a flawless aesthetic—and not one of them had a clue I was sick.

It wasn't because I had done such a stellar job applying my concealer—although that *did* help. Nobody knew because I had my own notable glam squad helping me maintain my looks during cancer treatment. I had Ted Gibson telling me how to brush my thinning hair without pulling out any additional strands. I had Dr. Brian Kantor (the dentist for 50 Cent, the New York Knicks, and Penelope Cruz) keeping me stocked up on rinses to prevent the mouth sores chemo normally caused. And I had Elle Gerstein, JLo's manicurist, giving me tips on how to keep my nails from falling out. For every physical feature that could possibly be affected by cancer treatment, I had an expert in that specialty on speed dial. And I called every one of them.

If I hadn't been a beauty director with such incredible sources, I wouldn't have been able to show up at the party looking so good, so "normal." Like any good reporter, I had done research before I started treatment but there wasn't one book, one website, one resource that had all the information I needed on how to maintain my skin, hair, nails, mouth—and even my vajajay—during cancer treatment.

For cancer patients, it's often considered taboo to care about your looks when you should be focused on fighting for your life. While it was important to keep perspective on the health goals at hand, looking good, for me, was equally vital to my recovery. It

The fact of the matter is beauty treatments are an adjunct therapy to cancer treatments. If you look good, you feel better. Even when I was feeling like shit—if I resembled a hint of my 'normal self,' it helped me get out of bed and power through the day. They say there are more important things in life than beauty and fashion but I'm here to tell you that they are just as important—if not more so—when you are sick. And why should anyone have to choose between their health or their beauty? They shouldn't—and don't—have to. The two are not mutually exclusive.

helped me stay positive and focused on living, rather than being sick and all the possible negative outcomes that can come of it.

I can't tell you how many times I faced scrutiny when I would inquire or talk about the aesthetic elements and side effects of my treatment. But why is it so wrong to care? Why are cancer patients made to feel vain if they want their mastectomy reconstruction results to look and feel like real breasts, or ask about losing their hair?

The fact of the matter is beauty treatments *are* an adjunct therapy to cancer treatments. If you look good, you feel better. Even when I was feeling like shit—if I resembled a hint of my "normal self," it helped me get out of bed and power through the day. They say there are more important things in life than beauty and fashion but I'm here to tell you that they are just as important—if not more so—when you are sick. And why should anyone have to choose between their health or their beauty? They shouldn't—and don't—have to. The two are not mutually exclusive.

Maybe it's because beauty came late in life to me, and I wasn't ready to give it up so fast. Growing up, I was a chubby redheaded child with a face full of freckles and a precocious personality. By high school, I had discovered my inner rebel thanks to the Sex Pistols. And I did my best to channel Johnny Rotten with a neon-orange bi-level bob, ten-hole Dr. Martens, and ripped clothes held together with safety pins. I also shared his pimply skin problem too, which didn't win me any boyfriends. By college, Madonna was my idol, so naturally push-up bras became my go-to fashion statement. I didn't have the bust for them, but I wore them like they were my job. When I took a gig as "shooter girl" doling out shots of tequila and vodka at the Wave, a nightclub on Long Beach Island, bustiers became my uniform. It was then that I realized the power of boobs and fashion. When I graduated, I landed a job as editorial assistant in the newsroom of my hometown paper. I worked the news desk typing up the fire calls, police blotter, and obituaries. While I knew all the juicy scoops in town, I longed for a more glamorous role. On the night

JLo wore that infamous slit dress to the MTV Video Music Awards, I scored an interview with the designer, Donatella Versace, and wrote up the story on deadline. It was selected as the cover. Two days later, I was promoted to the coveted job of fashion columnist.

While I loved fashion, it always felt a little cliquey to me. If you weren't a size two or rolling in money, there were certain things that would always be off-limits. *But beauty is democratic*. Obsessed with Beyoncé's limited edition Chanel bag? Good luck getting one. Love her smoky eye shadow? The look was easy to achieve—by anyone, on any budget. When I became a beauty director at a national magazine, I got to interview all the greats in the beauty world. I listened to their tips and tricks and then put them to work at home. In just a few years, I transformed into a full-fledged glamour girl. And it was just as I was feeling like I was coming into my own, achieving my potential fabulousness, that I was diagnosed with cancer. Talk about bad timing.

For the one in eight women who are diagnosed with breast cancer every year; the one in seventeen women diagnosed with lung cancer; or one in twenty-three who will be diagnosed with colorectal cancer, most of us don't know how to adjust our beauty routines during surgery, treatment, and life after. Most of us don't know what type of wig to shop for. Most don't know how to care for our skin when it's undergoing intense radiation. Why? Because there has never been a book dedicated to comprehensive beauty advice for cancer patients. Until now.

Pretty Sick: The Beauty Guide for Women with Cancer is my way of paying forward all the amazing advice, tips, and tricks that I received during my battle with breast cancer. That intel helped me look and feel better during the darkest days of my life. My hope is that by paving the way, it makes the journey less bumpy for you.

XO,
Caitlin

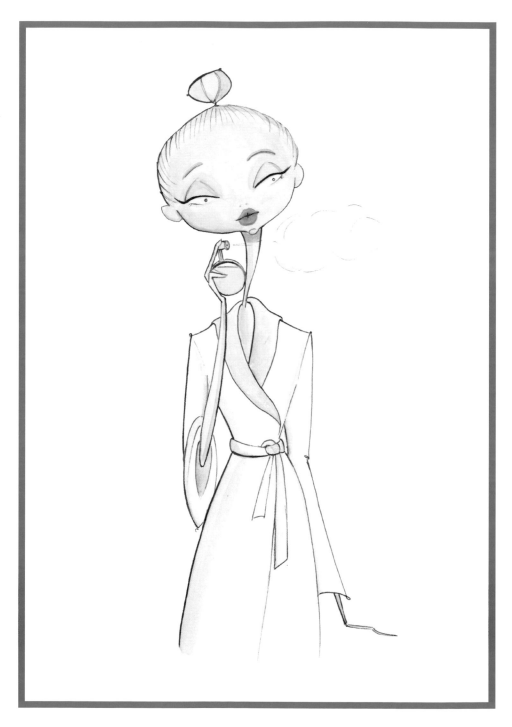

CHAPTER 1

THIS STINKS!

···

how treatment affects your sense of smell

···

Smell. I know this is the *last* thing you are probably thinking about right now. But as a cancer survivor, and former beauty director, it's the *first* thing I'm going to ask you to consider. Here's why:

From this point forward, every minute of this journey you are now on is going to be captured forever in your brain by your sense of smell. Mundane moments, even fleeting seconds, that you will most likely forget: sitting in the chemo suite with a drip in your arm; putting your wig on in the morning; taking a shower weeks after surgery—will be stored in your mind like a Polaroid picture by your sense of smell. One familiar whiff—and bam!—you will be transported back to any of these moments by your sense of smell. Memories, emotions, will feel as raw and real as they did when you first lived them. This phenomenon is called "scent memory."

Scent memory is a normal—yet unique—occurrence that we've all experienced: the aroma of fresh peeled apples brings you back to baking with your grandma; a breeze of lilac and you're playing again in the yard of your childhood home; a specific hair spray reminds you of prom night twenty years ago. Over half of the patients in chemotherapy treatment will experience temporary changes to their sense of smell. Those having radiation therapy for head and neck cancers can also experience a reduced or heightened sense of smell. This change of sense can trigger powerful memories months and years down the road.

So why am I telling you this? What does this have to do with cancer and your beauty regimen? *A lot* actually. I'm going to share a story to explain why.

A year before I was diagnosed with breast cancer, I had major back surgery. During that time, I used all of my regular skin care products. Why wouldn't I, right? A year later—after a rotation of different cleansers, serums, and toners—I came back to that same La Prairie face cream that I had used during my recovery from surgery. Instantly, I started having flashbacks to the days when I was out of work on disability, and, in essence, learning how to walk again. It was one of the most difficult times in my life and the memories brought up by the smell of that face cream made me feel depressed and helpless all over again. The emotions were so terrible, so tangible, I felt like I was reliving the whole experience.

Obviously, I didn't want a reoccurrence of this during my battle with breast cancer. So, after my initial doctors appointments and a week before my first surgery, I switched out all my staple (and favorite) beauty products. Instead of opting for inexpensive drugstore replacements, I decided to be a bit indulgent and choose some really luxurious products. I mean, why not? The road ahead was going to suck. This was the least I could do to pamper myself both emotionally and physically. I stocked up on La Mer moisturizer, Rodin Olio Lusso body oil, and Fresh Hesperides Grapefruit Bath & Shower Gel. I figured that the high-end ingredients would be essential in healing my ravaged skin and I wouldn't miss the hefty price tags if the smells reminded me of this shitty time in my life.

So, why does our sense of smell change?

"One theory is that a number of chemotherapeutic agents alter cell turnover in the olfactory pathway, the olfactory hypothelium, or the cells at the top of the nose," says Dr. Richard Doty, the director of

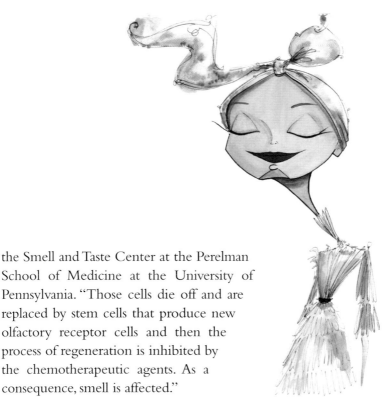

the Smell and Taste Center at the Perelman School of Medicine at the University of Pennsylvania. "Those cells die off and are replaced by stem cells that produce new olfactory receptor cells and then the process of regeneration is inhibited by the chemotherapeutic agents. As a consequence, smell is affected."

> ## Now *is the time to shelve your favorite beauty products.*

Specific chemotherapy drugs responsible for affecting smell include: carboplatin, cisplatin, cyclophosphamide, dacarbazine, dactinomycin, doxorubicin, 5-fluorouracil, levamisole, mechlorethamine, methotrexate, paclitaxel, and vincristine.

In her book *The Scent of Desire*, Dr. Rachel Herz, one of the leading experts in the psychology of smell, discusses the very realness of this phenomenon. "More than any other sensory experience, fragrances have the ability to trigger our emotions: to fill us with joy and rage, to bring us to tears and to make our hearts ache, to incite us with terror, and to titillate our desires." Herz goes on to write how many New Yorkers who survived the attacks on the World Trade Center on September 11, 2001, have this experience whenever they smell anything charred or dusty. She adds one stunning fact that can't be ignored. "Not only do odors trigger emotions, they can *become* emotions." How is this possible? The reason is this: No other sensory system (sight, taste, touch, hearing) makes direct contact with the amygdala, the area of the brain where emotion and emotional memory is processed and the hippocampus, where associative learning takes place. Because of this, Herz writes, "odors can literally be transformed into emotions through association and then act as proxies for emotions themselves, influencing how we feel, how we think and how we act." The two are fundamentally interconnected while being independently functional.

Studies show that children and adults exposed to "frustration-associated odors" during tests were less creative and motivated to solve the problems compared to their peers who weren't exposed and ultimately successful at the tasks presented. Just think about the effect a scent memory—linked to the day of your surgery, wig shopping, or your radiation treatments—could do to your positive attitude and recovery process. It can be life-altering, I will tell you that.

Here's the thing: most beauty products—even the unscented ones—have a smell. And because of that, they aren't exempt from scent memories. So, here's my advice:

Now is the time to shelve your favorite beauty products.

This includes obvious items like your perfume and body lotion but it also applies to things you normally won't think twice about, like toothpaste and hand wash. Making this swap early—as close to the day of your diagnosis as possible—will prevent them from having any connection to your cancer. After all your treatments and surgeries are over, you can swap your favorites back in. But during this time, treat yourself to a few items you wouldn't normally splurge on. You deserve it—and so does your body!

perfume: to spritz or *not* to spritz

In many ways, perfume tells the story of a person's life. For me, each chapter of my life is defined by the perfume I was wearing at the time. In high school I wore Giorgio Beverly Hills. In college, it was Elizabeth Arden's Red. For my first job I wore YSL's Opium a scent I thought was mature and sophisticated. The day I was offered the beauty director position, I had traces of Jo Malone Orange Blossom lingering on my wrists and neck. Today, I'm all about Tom Ford Private Blend. For most women—and many men—perfume helps us project to the world who we aspire to be. This is certainly true for me. So, when I was sick, I didn't want to give that up. I still wanted to smell feminine, sexy—like my (regular) self. I wanted, no, *needed*, that element of normalcy and happiness.

Studies show that the very existence of scent elevates one's mood. People who have lost their ability to smell—no matter what the cause—are more likely to experience depression. So, while it can be tricky for cancer patients to use products with fragrance, if you're anything like me, it's still very important to have some wafting around. So, if you are going to wear perfume, my advice is that you set aside your signature scent and find a temporary replacement.

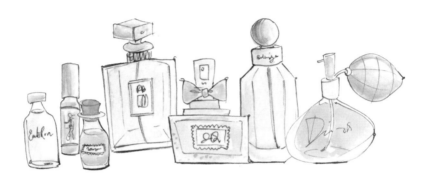

Now I know what you're going to say: You've worn the same fragrance for the last ten years. It's your absolute favorite and everyone knows when you enter a room by the gorgeous aroma that trails behind you. This is precisely why you *don't* want to wear it now. Besides the fact that you don't want to create cancer-affiliated scent memories, the changing chemicals in your skin will most likely cause the perfume to produce a different smell than what you are used to. "I think this is essential information for patients who are being treated," says Dr. Avery Gilbert, psychologist from the University of Pennsylvania and author of *What the Nose Knows: The Science of Scent in Everyday Life*. "It's very important to shelve your favorite fragrance for a while, so that you don't link it to the negative aspect of the experience." Instead, choose a backup blend that you love almost as much but could stand to live without in the long run. Here's how to do just that...

determine your skin's sensitivity

The first thing you want to do is evaluate how sensitive your skin is to determine the concentration that it can handle. Granted, this may change once chemotherapy or radiation treatments commence but it will give you a baseline gauge for how reactive your skin is and might be. If your skin tends to get itchy, red, or irritated from the cold weather, allergies, or a sweat-filled workout—that indicates it could be supersensitive once you are in the thick of treatment. "Fragrances are categorized by the range of concentration that they fall into," says Lisa Lewis, senior vice president and Fragrance Academy Director at Givaudan, global leader in the creation of fragrance and flavors. The Swiss-based company is behind some of the most iconic and best-selling fragrances including Calvin Klein Obsession, Dior J'adore, Angel by Thierry Mugler, Gucci Guilty, and Dolce & Gabbana—to name a few. "Going from a lower concentration to a higher concentration you have: body mists/splash, eau de toilette, perfume/parfum, and then essential oils."

start light, finish strong

If your skin seems a little sensitive but you still want to wear a scent, it's safest to try a body mist or splash first. These contain the lowest concentration of fragrance, making them the mildest option and the fastest to evaporate in the skin, hence the least irritating. My advice: Do a patch test on a hidden part of your body and see how your skin fares. If no reaction occurs, you can probably handle a more concentrated fragrance like an eau de toilette. If an eau de toilette is no problem, move on to perfume. You will only know by giving it a test run.

spray, delay, then decide

Selecting a "swap in" fragrance when your skin and sense of smell are changing can be challenging. The pH of your skin, your body chemistry, has a direct impact on how a fragrance smells. Conversely, the change in the mucous membranes of your nose will affect how you interpret that smell. So, it's important to test potential candidates on your skin before making a decision. "You should give a fragrance an hour to really experience it," says Lewis. "When you first spray, you get the top notes. Then, over the next ten to thirty minutes is what we call the mid-notes. Followed by the residual, the dry down, which is what lingers on your skin." That ending aroma often smells completely different from how it started, so it's important to give it time to diffuse completely before breaking out the benjamins.

give it time, before you rewind

When can you go back to wearing your oldie but goodie? The earliest would be one month after chemo ends. "The figures given for the complete turnover of the cells in the nose is something in the order of thirty to thirty-five days," says Dr. Gilbert. His advice: "Because cell turnover has been slowed down or knocked down a bit, it might take a little bit more time. Two months would be the safe waiting time to bring back your signature scent or the original brands you used to use."

scentsational notes

Scent has the amazing ability to change how we feel—so why not harness that to enhance your mojo? When you're shopping for a new fragrance, consider the notes it contains. Over the last two decades, Givaudan and International Flavors & Fragrance (among others) have studied the subjective and physiological effects of aromas and fragrances on emotions via "mood mapping." "There are studies about how different fragrances can impact different moods and that can be extremely effective for patients," says Lewis, whose mother is a two-time breast cancer survivor. Below are some notes that work wonders for your well-being.

uplifting

Need a quick pick-me-up? Instead of grabbing a coffee, spritz a citrus-based scent instead! Notes including *orange*, *grapefruit*, *bergamot*, and *lemon* are energizing. So are certain florals. A study conducted in 2010 revealed that the tiny flower *jasmine* could help relieve depressive thoughts and increase alertness with one whiff!

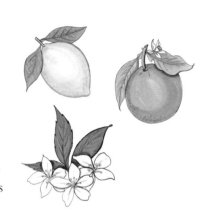

soothing

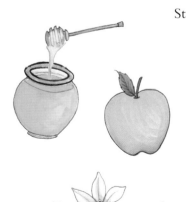

Studies show that if you are looking to attract a mate you should select a fragrance with gourmand notes including *honey*, *chocolate*, and *vanilla*, which have aphrodisiacal powers. (Men think they are absolutely scrumptious!) But they also have the ability to calm the nerves. This capability also extends to warmer notes like *amber* (which smells like vanilla) and *sandalwood*. But there is one surprising scent that acts like an air-based Xanax: *green apple*. During a control panel conducted in 2008, the scent helped control feelings of anxiety during stressful moments and provided a noticeable reduction in headaches including migraines. Apparently, "An apple a day keeps the doctor away" isn't just some stupid expression…

relaxing

There's a reason why **lavender** oil is used in almost every spa—it's well documented for easing both the mind and body. But did you know that green, leafy notes do too? Researchers in Australia found that a chemical released by newly mown **grass** makes people more joyful and relaxed. **Pine** also has some relaxing powers. A study conducted at Japan's Kyoto University examined the Japanese custom of strolling in the forest, known as shinrin-yoku or "forest bathing." On the days participants walked through the pine-filled woods, their levels of depression and anxiety were significantly reduced. Here's my advice for those who celebrate Christmas: The next time your relatives are coming over for the holidays, it might be wise to get a *real* pine tree…

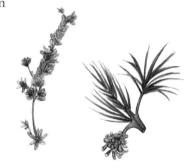

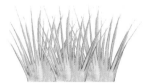

a word about *oils*

Fragrance or perfume oils are typically made with essential oils. Because the scent is more concentrated, it also tends to be more irritating on the skin. Besides the potential to cause headaches and nausea, they can also prompt hives, rashes, and sores. For those with estrogen-positive cancers, like myself, there are some oils that should be avoided. These essential oils contain phytoestrogens that can mimic estrogen in the body, enhance the effects of estrogen, or cause symptoms of estrogen depletion—any of which may result in a hormonal imbalance. While the levels are probably nothing to worry about in dab-sized applications, it's important to be informed and aware of any potential side effects they could cause. Three oils are especially known to exaggerate changes in estrogen levels: lavender, rosemary, and tea tree oil. Others to avoid include clove, chamomile, licorice, oregano, peppermint, nutmeg, thyme, sage, and verbena.

fragrance-free

With all the products we use every day—from hand wash to hair spray—it's almost impossible to use all fragrance-free beauty products. Finding a shampoo without a "fresh" scent is tough! But your health is worth the hunt. When shopping, labels can often be misleading. Terms like "hypoallergenic," "natural," and "organic" don't necessarily mean they are fragrance-free or gentle. You have to read the ingredient list and give the product a good whiff to know for sure. Some products are scented with fruit or herb extracts and those are generally natural and nonirritating. Choosing scent-free beauty products is the safer route and will help keep your skin smooth, supple, and rash-free. An extensive list of brands and specific scent-free products can be found in Chapter 3 (page 67). Use that list as a guide for what products to buy and use while in treatment.

where to wear your fragrance

Unless you've been hiding under a rock, you probably know that the pulse points of the body—wrists, neck, bend of the arm, behind the knees, temples, ankles—are the best places to apply perfume. These areas are where the main arteries of the body stream with warm blood, which heats the skin and helps diffuse a fragrance. For those who don't have any skin sensitivities or changes in scent—go wild! But those of you who are experiencing either issue should be more strategic in where and how you apply fragrance. Here are some non–pulse point options:

mist your clothes

"People who have sensitive skin but still want to smell good should spray their garments," advises Lewis. Spritzing your clothes before you put them on ensures the fragrance doesn't come in contact with your skin. It's important to note that chemicals used to create fragrances can be damaging to certain fabrics—so don't douse your duds. An airy mist is all you need.

scent your strands

Fragrance molecules absorb quickly into hair fibers, which is why some people believe it's a better place than skin to apply scent. Because the alcohol content in fragrance can be drying, instead of spraying directly onto strands, mist it onto a brush or comb, then run it through the hair. My cancer buddy Kristen used to apply her perfume to the ends of her wig. The placement on her bob made it smell like she was wearing fragrance on her neck. I still think this is a genius trick.

spritz unexpected spots

If your skin isn't sensitive but your nose is, applying on your neck isn't the best area. Instead, opt for places farther from your face—like the wrist and ankles. Don't worry that you won't whiff it—heat rises. Some fragrance experts also advise wearing your scent on unexpected areas of the body that throw heat—like the middle of the back and behind the knees.

be *aware* of the *air* you *share*

One tip I want to end on is something I think is of equal importance to the information above…Just because you like your perfume, eau de toilette, or fragrance oil, doesn't mean everybody does. This is especially true in hospitals and chemo suites where patients are highly susceptible to smells. Most cancer institutes have a no-perfume policy out of courtesy to their patients. Cancer or no cancer— you should always be mindful of where you are going and whom you will be around before you start spritzing. As a former beauty director, when I interviewed the leading perfumers and "noses" in the industry, all of them had one discriminating rule about applying scent: Fragrance is an intimate experience. It should not permeate around you. Instead, it should require another to lean in—for a kiss or a hug—to be revealed. I completely agree. This creates an air of mystery that is intriguing and sexy while being respectful to those around you.

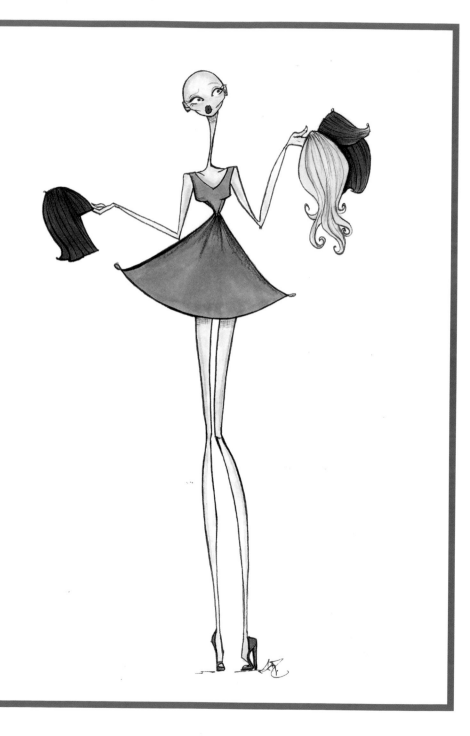

CHAPTER 2
THE MANE EVENT

hair today, gone tomorrow

I always think it's funny that a pink ribbon is the symbol for breast cancer. So pretty. So feminine. So delicate. To me, it connotes the opposite feelings—both emotionally and physically—of the toll this disease takes. Don't get me wrong; I get the reasoning behind it. As a beauty director who was in charge of our magazine's annual October Breast Cancer Awareness issues, I fully understand the power of its positive branding. But as a cancer survivor, it seems a bit, well, trite. Personally, I think the symbol should have been a bit more honest—and humorous (right about now we all need more of that, right?). If anybody had asked me,

I would have picked something like the Twitter egg—you know, that faceless, hairless, default profile picture it assigns everybody before they upload their own photo. Why? Well, when you think of cancer, what image comes to mind first? A bald head—that's what! When you see a person without hair—walking down the street, shopping for clothes, entering a restaurant—you know *instantly* they are battling the Big C.

"Our images of cancer come more from the treatment of the disease, than the disease itself," says Dr. Mindy Greenstein, psycho-oncologist and clinical psychologist who is a consultant to the psychiatry department at Memorial Sloan Kettering. She is also a breast cancer survivor. "When people think of cancer, they think of baldness, for instance. But cancer doesn't do that. Chemo does that."

For cancer patients who find themselves on the opposite end of those knowing stares, it drives home the realness of this crappy disease. So a pink ribbon's got nothing on a hairless head. A bald head really is the symbol of cancer. There is no escaping that truth. And while doctors and patients both know hair loss is a probable—or inevitable—side effect of cancer treatment, it is often the first question those newly diagnosed ask their oncologists: "Am I going to lose my hair?"

I wasn't any different.

For as long as I can remember, my mother always used to tell me: "Your hair is your asset." While my sisters were born with perfect features and killer bodies, I had been blessed with long, thick, wavy locks. When I curled my hair, it would look like something out of an Herbal Essence commercial. Bouncy, shiny, and super sexy. Gisele had nothing on me (okay, minus her flawless face and *that* body…) But my hair really was gorgeous. So when I had that chemo convo, I obviously freaked out at the thought of losing the one thing—the main thing—that made me look and feel beautiful: my hair.

Let's circle back for a bit…

I was diagnosed with breast cancer in July 2012. After a lumpectomy, my oncologist gave me the rundown of my pathology report and the various treatment options.

The tumor, located in my right breast, was just under one centimeter, well differentiated, and HER2 negative. The Oncotype DX test, which analyzes the genes of the cancer and determines its probable recurrence rate, was eighteen—the first number in the middle range. It was the best scenario of a bad situation. While my doctors told me I would have to have radiation to kill any remaining cancer cells still lurking in the breast tissue, they were on the fence about chemotherapy because of my low Onco score. I remember my oncologist, Dr. Clifford Hudis, saying to me, "It's up to you. But if you are the type of person that is going to be looking over your shoulder or if you think you'll regret having not done chemotherapy if the cancer comes back—then you should do it." Sold! I wanted the best chance of survival so I decided to do chemotherapy.

"The important thing to understand from a beauty standpoint, is that the chemo goes directly to the fast-growing cells in your body because cancer is totally out-of-control, rapidly growing cells. But there are other rapidly growing cells in your body, for instance, your skin, hair follicles, nails. That's why you lose your hair," says Joan Lunden, legendary newswoman, former host of *Good Morning America,* and author of the *New York Times* best-selling memoir *Had I Known* about her battle and survival with stage II triple negative breast cancer. "And you lose it much faster than you think—in seven to fourteen days." She is quick to add, "By the way, let's just tell women—you lose your hair *everywhere*. I mean, you don't have hair on your arm, or your legs or anywhere else. It's basically like a bikini wax you don't have to pay for." Silver linings, ladies. Silver linings.

While I knew I was in good hands and that my doctors had things under control—it was the thought of losing my hair that was immediately concerning. "It is *so* distressing," shares Joan. I was especially freaked out about the thought of losing my eyelashes and eyebrows. As sucky as it is to lose your hair—and it IS really sucky—it IS also manageable. You get a stylish wig or wear some really fun hats or colorful scarves. You can even decorate a bald head with Swarovski crystals! The bottom line: You can cover or accessorize a bald head. Losing your eyebrows and eyelashes—that's a totally different situation. Since I was still working full-time at the magazine, I was really nervous that my eyebrow-less face would be a telltale sign that I was sick. I didn't want to feel like I was at a professional disadvantage. But being sick, I clearly was. *I* knew I was sick but I didn't need *everybody* else to. I knew losing my hair and my eyebrows would expose me. And it does. That is the harsh reality. I was going to have to suck it up and deal with it. But I was going to do it stylishly.

Before the moment of my diagnosis, I had never had to think about what my hair meant to me. Sure, I had had my fair share of bad haircuts and dye jobs: the Johnny Rotten orange bi-level I wore sophomore year in high school; the jet-black caesar I got at the height of my club kids days in the early nineties; the bleached blond straggly layers I wore when channeling Madonna during college. But no matter how bad or how much I regretted a cut or color—I never let it bum me out. My sister, Siobhan, would cry after every haircut. I thought she was nuts. She would ask for a dramatic cut and then sob the minute it was done. I felt terrible for her stylist. I just never cared that much about my hair—until I was losing it. It was only then that I quickly realized how attached I was and how much I identified myself through my long, wavy strands.

"I don't think most people realize the magnitude of what hair means," says Ted Gibson, stylist to the most beautiful actresses in the world including Angelina Jolie, Ashley Greene, Cameron Diaz, Lupita Nyong'o, Ariana Grande, Debra Messing, and Taylor Schilling. "It's hard to explain how important it is but I think it's more important than just about anything else in a woman's life. And I know because I see it. When a woman sits in my chair—she comes in one way and leaves a totally different woman. Hair changes everything."

#truth

When I was first diagnosed, Ted was the first person I turned to to help me face my soon-to-be-bald situation head-on. The best advice he gave me at that time, which he repeated again for this book, was this: "Take control." In a serious tone, he explains that thought, "Being prepared with a plan on how to handle your hair loss is better than waiting until the last moment and reacting to it happening."

ted's *tips* for handling your hair loss
have a game plan

The first thing you want to do is to go shopping for a wig while you still have hair. You might only a have a few days to go shopping before your chemo begins; however, it's important for the wig specialist to see what your hair looks like while you have it. More on this later…

get a *buzz*-worthy look

One trend to try before breaking out the buzzers: hair tattoos! "It sounds scary, like getting an actual tattoo, but that's not the case," says *New York Times* Life Interrupted columnist Suleika Jaouad, who was diagnosed with aggressive myeloid leukemia at age twenty-two. "I went to this funky basement barbershop called Astor Place Hair in lower Manhattan and I would have the barber groove designs into my hair with his clipper. For me, it was a way to take an unfortunate situation and turn it into something that felt stylish and made me feel beautiful. I remember when I walked out of the barbershop a construction worker whistled at me and said 'Awesome hair!' That was the first comment anyone had made about my hair since my diagnosis that wasn't cancer-related. It felt good to own that and to turn my head into a canvas and not something that represented me as a sick person."

don't wait for your hair to fall out. cut that shizz!!!

After selecting a wig, cut your hair short. "Losing your hair is a very traumatic thing," says Ted. "However, it's inevitable when going through this aggressive type of treatment. Cutting your hair, before it starts to fall out in patches, gives you a sense of control. It can be devastating to see hair falling out. So, cutting it—in stages or even just going short—will help minimize how upsetting that can be."

Joan agrees. "It is so emotionally trying when the hair starts coming out. It will come out in your hands, it'll be on your pillow, and it will come out in clumps in your brush," she shares. "That's why I really recommend getting in front of it. I had gone to the spa in the salon to get a spray tan and I asked, 'Is there someone here who can shave my head? I am going to lose my hair in like a week so I'd rather have a head-to-toe spray tan.' There's nothing worse than a bald head, than a pink bald head!"

In all aspects of my life I have one mantra: "Go big or go home." This applies to everything in my life: eyelashes, nails, handbags, heels—you know, the things that matter. So, when faced with the fact that I was going to lose my hair, I decided to take Ted's advice and cut it short. The style I wanted was Rihanna's pompadour. Remember that edgy crop she rocked? Buzzed on the sides, long on the top. I was *ob-sessed* with that style. I had actually flirted with the idea of getting that cut even before I got sick but I never had the balls to do it. I was sure—with my square (aka masculine) jawline and flat chest—that I would look like a boy. But when cancer entered the picture, I actually got excited at the thought of wearing such a bold, fashion-forward cut. During some dark days, it gave me something to look forward to and to have fun with.

This approach, of having a game plan, is so empowering. And in many ways, it will be your saving grace. It was for my friend, Elena Tavarez, a second-generation breast cancer survivor and hairstylist at Cutler Salon in New York City's Soho. Before her diagnosis, Elena was not only known for creating beautiful hair on other people—she was also known for *her* hair: long, smooth chocolate-brown locks that fell to her waist and rarely required styling to look absolutely stunning. "It was my *thing* and it was gorgeous," she recalls. "But after the nurse told me I was going to lose my hair, I said, 'Fuck this! I'm just going to cut my hair. I'm going to be in charge of this.'"

For many women, like Elena and me, hair is a tangible memory. We associate and remember life events by what our hair looked like at those times. Just look at pictures from your prom, college, or wedding—your hairstyle speaks volumes about what was happening in your life, in pop culture, in fashion. So, for Elena—whose whole world revolves around hair—making the decision to cut it short

> **During the third and fourth stages of sleep (also known as slow-wave or deep-sleep phases), the body heals itself. It is this rest and recovery phase that will enable your body to stay strong during treatment. So don't skip on sleep—or the head massages that will lead to it.**

was equal parts ballsy and brave. "For me, it became about having a cute hairstyle rather than a connection to my cancer," she says of her decision to chop it into a bob. "A few weeks after my chemo treatments began and my hair began to fall out, I cut it again into a cute pixie." Eventually, she broke out the buzzer. But up until that moment, she was having fun with her new styles, rather than focusing on the sadness of the situation. "When I finally buzzed it off, I was like, okay, well, that's done. Now I can just move on to the next thing." The gradual goodbye was her way of dealing with and accepting her diagnosis. While the plan was to send her cut hair to Locks of Love they remain—to this day—in her desk in a ziplock bag. "I never thought I was attached to my hair," she reflects. "Initially, I just thought I wasn't ready. But I still just can't seem to let it go." This revelation speaks to how most of us feel about our hair. It is part of who we are and we have a deep connection to it beyond just the physical.

As it turns out, I never got the Rihanna cut. On the day of my appointment, I was literally leaving my office to go to the salon when I got a phone call. It was from a friend who had gotten me an appointment with Dr. Clifford Hudis, the then chief of breast medicine at Memorial Sloan Kettering, whom I had been waitlisted to see. Obviously, I chose to go to *that* appointment instead. And during that meeting he informed me that the chemo regimen he was going to put me on was only going to cause "hair thinning"—not hair loss. I had dodged a bullet. Or in this case, buzzers. But either way, I still wasn't out of the woods.

For those of us lucky enough to keep some of our hair during treatment—whether from cold caps (more on this on page 59) or varying chemo regimens, there are a few things you can do to help reduce the stress on the hair and prolong its placement. Some of the tips and information I am about to share will even apply to those who are in the shedding stage before full hair loss.

talk about *touchy*

Let's start by talking about touching your head. Yes, *touching* your head. This may sound odd, but when I started chemo, I was so nervous that anything that came into contact with my head would make my hair fall out. If anyone made a fast motion around me, I would pull out my best *Karate Kid* moves. The fear became so great that I wouldn't touch my scalp, wouldn't brush my hair; I barely even washed it. I figured the less pressure on the follicle, the more hair I would keep in my head. This is delusional, of course. And actually the complete opposite of what you should do.

"You can't prevent the hair that is going to fall out from falling out. Those follicles are dead," says Ted. "But you can massage the scalp to stimulate blood flow to the live follicles, which will make the hair that remains stronger and healthier." Massage also has some additional benefits. According to ancient Ayurvedic practices, massage encourages relaxation and sleep. This may sound irrelevant but a good night's sleep is probably *the* best gift you can give yourself right now. Why?

During the third and fourth stages of sleep (also known as slow-wave or deep-sleep phases), the body heals itself. It is this rest and recovery phase that will enable your body to stay strong during treatment. So don't skip on sleep—or the head massages that *will* lead to it.

You can do this on yourself but it can be equally beneficial and a way to bond with a loved one—if they do it on you. Here's a quick how-to:

how to give good head (massage)

1   Place your hands on either side of your head with the fingertips meeting in the center of the forehead and the thumbs on your temples.

2   Use your fingers to apply pressure to this spot on your forehead while circulating the thumbs on the temples. Then circulate your fingers. Release the pressure, then shift your fingers farther up toward the hairline. Then reapply pressure and circulate your fingers on the scalp.

3   Repeat until your fingers are three-quarters back on the top of your head. Your thumbs will be positioned at the top of the ears and the fingers on the center of the scalp. This spot is the governor vessel 20 acupoint. This pressure point is believed to help balance the yin and yang of the body, to encourage sleep, and to sharpen mental facilities. When you reach this spot, spend an extra, thoughtful moment applying pressure.

4 Continue until you reach the nape of the neck. When there, begin the steps in reverse, moving hands back to their starting position at the forehead.

brusha-*brusha*-brusha

While having *any* hair during chemo is a blessing, I totally empathize with those of you who are shedding and trying to preserve hair with cold caps (more on them later, page 59). In many ways, shedding is more stressful than losing your hair altogether because you are constantly worrying about the amount of hair you've lost. But rather than freaking out about it, I am going to give you tips on the best ways to care for your hair while you have it. This way, you can focus your energy toward getting healthy again.

So, let's start with the basics.

The benefit of a comb is that it doesn't pull or add pressure to the fragile hair follicles. Ted and I both agree that a comb is the best option to use while hair is thinning. It's important to keep hair from matting or getting knotty so that you don't have to wrestle and pull on it when that happens. I prefer a wide-tooth, wooden comb because it won't snap the hair and does not create static electricity. Wood is also hypoallergenic, which may sound ridiculous when talking about a comb, but many of the plastic brushes are coated in chemicals that could be irritating for those with sensitive scalps or skin. I really like Long Time Sun Apparel combs (www.longtime sunapparel.com), which have an all-natural beeswax or linseed oil coating to protect the wood. Hair is more fragile, and heavier, when wet, so it's best to comb and detangle hair when it is dry—before getting in the shower.

how to comb delicate hair

1   Take your nondominant hand and lay it flat against your head, about two inches below the roots. (I position my fingers facing the back of the head, with the wrist close to the hairline—but do it whichever way is most comfortable for you.)

2   Hold hand firmly without tugging on the hair. The point of this is to use your hand to hold the hair in place so it doesn't move or tug on the roots when combing.

3   Take the comb in the opposite hand and place it in the hair directly below your hand.

4   Gingerly glide the comb through to the ends.

5   Move hand to next section of hair and repeat until the entire head is combed.

it's a *wash!*

Now that we've discussed how to brush your hair, let's chat about washing it. Showering was always a worrisome situation for me because it meant coming face-to-face with the tangible reality of my hair loss. My friend Vivienne (not her real name), who was losing her hair at the same time, used to count each strand that fell out. I don't recommend this move. It sent her over the edge. Understandably. But why torture yourself? There isn't enough Xanax in the world for that. Plus, bottom line: it's hair. It *will* grow back.

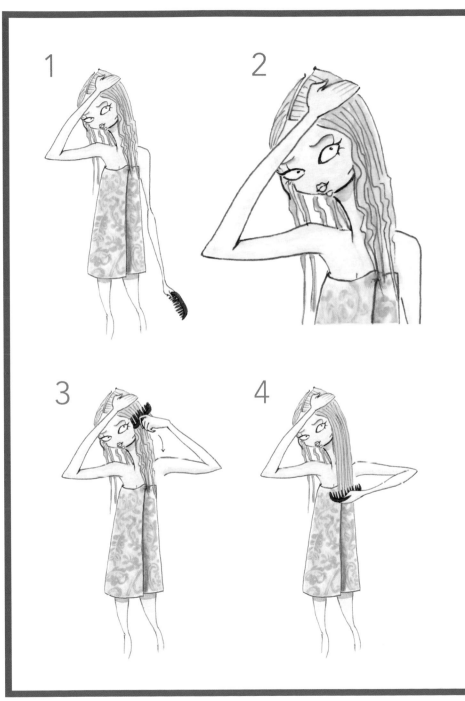

use sulfate-free shampoos

Skin gets supersensitive, itchy, and prone to hives during treatment. Since the scalp is skin, you're going to want to make sure you are using a sulfate-free shampoo and conditioner. Here's why: Sulfates are mineral salts containing sulfur. Many hair products are formulated with sulfates because they help create a rich lather. Apparently, people love a halo of foam on their heads while they shower. While sulfates are not dangerous, they are extremely drying. They also cause scalp irritations, breakouts, split ends, frizz, and give skin and hair a dull appearance. While this might not be a big deal for the average, "healthy" person, the side effects of sulfates can be very irritating for someone whose skin is sensitive from chemo or radiation treatments. When shopping for shampoo, make sure to read the ingredient list so that you can avoid them. Sulfates appear on labels by a number of names, including: sodium laurel sulfate, sodium laureth sulfate, and sodium lauryl sulfate.

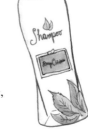

choose mild formulas

Choose a "hydrating" or "moisturizing" formula containing essential oils and fatty acids, such as jojoba, almond, argan, coconut, or sesame oils. These ingredients will ensure your scalp and skin are clean *and* moisturized. Avoid "clarifying" or "daily" shampoos, as they are harsh on the skin and hair.

limit how often you wash

Putting a limit on how many times a week you shampoo will be helpful. Twice a week is ideal. This gives the natural oils from your scalp time to distribute through the hair, conditioning strands in the process. Frequent cleaning actually strips away those key humectants.

That's counterintuitive when your skin and hair needs as much moisture as possible.

styling your strands

As I mentioned before, I was working full-time during my treatment. As a beauty director, I felt an extra level of pressure to look not only healthy but attractive as well. This is a feat on an average day. So, throw sickness into the mix and I'm sure you can imagine what a struggle it was. Many days, all I wanted to do was throw my hair up in a topknot but couldn't because I didn't want to pull on the follicles. The good news is that just because the styling options are limited, that doesn't mean having a good hair day is hopeless. Ted shares his key styling tips:

little changes make a big difference

"Even if you do something a little bit differently—like changing the part—it can create a whole new look," says Ted. Per his suggestion, I would change my part two or three times a week because that gave me a variety of looks. Just switch it up!

beachy texture is best

Beachy texture is the best type of curl/wave to wear because it is *supposed* to look a little messy. That's what makes it so effortless and wearable. It's also an easy texture to create without putting stress on the hair or follicles. At night, after showering, I would let my hair air dry. When it was still a little damp, I would create three loose braids (one on the left side, one on the right and one in the back). I would start the braid just above ear level and then loosely weave it down to the ends—securing it with a no-grip elastic band (my favorites are from Goody). By morning, the braids would be dry and when I took them out—voilà!—flirty, carefree waves.

easy is chic

There is nothing as eye-catching as a braid. They look intricate but are actually quite simple to create. I am also a big fan of twists as well. The point being: You don't have to do ornate styles or dramatic updos to look pretty. Occasionally, when I needed my hair to look more polished, I would use soft foam rollers. The downside is that it can take hours to dry (even with help from a blow-dryer). The upside is they are more gentle than styling tools like curling or flat irons and create a smooth curl that often lasts a few days. I used the large two-inch foam rollers so that I didn't end up looking like Shirley Temple, which I found out the hard way after using a smaller size.

no pressure please!

Any style that requires grippy accessories or tools should be a no-go while the hair is thinning. Ponytails, buns, topknots, sleek, flat-ironed strands—any style that requires tugging or pulling on the hair could result in hair loss. Better safe than sorry.

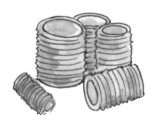

getting *wiggy* with it

Wigs. Drag queens might love 'em but for those of us that *have* to wear them…it's not so much fun. But it *can* be! You just have to get your head around the fact that wearing one is temporary. Right after I was diagnosed, when the doctors thought I would need to

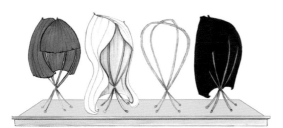

be on a stronger chemo regimen and would lose all my hair, I didn't let myself get upset about it. Instead, I was kinda excited—and I credit Wendy Williams for that. When I was a beauty director, I made a few appearances on *The Wendy Williams Show*. Every time I went on the show, Wendy was rocking a different wig and looked gorgeous. I loved how openly she talked about her wigs and hairpieces. She was the first national media personality who kept it real and, in the process, raised awareness (especially for white women) about wigs, wig maintenance, and just how much fun and useful they can be. When I was diagnosed, I decided I was going to channel Wendy. I wasn't going to cry over losing my hair—I was going to have fun finding a wig and look hot wearing it!

When it came to sharing advice for finding a wig, I thought there was no better person than Wendy to point us in the right direction. "Everyone wears fake hair these days," says the talk show host and media mogul during an interview in her glamorous New York City office. While most cancer patients use an easy on-off wig, it will be good for you to be familiar with the various options so that you don't get confused when shopping and know exactly what you want and need. Knowledge is power—or, in this case—prettiness.

wig *101:* the basics

There are two different types of "hair" used in wig-making: real and synthetic. Below are the pros and cons of each, which will help narrow down the option that is best suited for your look and lifestyle. In the long run, having a little intel will save you time, money, and bad hair days.

real hair wigs

A real hair wig is made from virgin human hair. Ninety percent of this hair comes from India and Asia. Virgin hair is hair that has never been damaged by chemical treatments including color, bleach, keratin, or perms. The benefit of a wig made with human hair is that it looks *really* real.

PROs:

It can be styled: A wig made with real hair can be heat styled just as if it was attached to your head. Want a beachy wave? Break out the curling iron. Want a sleek look? Reach for the blow-dryer or flat iron. When you can switch up your styles, it adds to the believability that it is your natural hair.

The part can be switched: With real hair wigs, the strands are individually sewn into the cap. This makes each hair look like it's growing from its own follicles. As a result, the cap resembles your scalp and gives you the freedom to play with the part.

It can be cut and colored: What makes wigs look, well, wiggy, is that they lack movement and the color tends to be either too shiny, too flat, or too stripy. A real hair wig can be cut and colored by your own stylist, who can add dimension and bounce that mimics your natural locks.

It is durable: That expression "You get what you pay for" is most applicable with the strength and quality of a wig made with real hair. The hairs are individually sewn into the cap, which promotes its quality and stability.

CONs:

It requires a lot of upkeep: A real hair wig will require the same maintenance as your own hair. The natural oils from your scalp, makeup, and any dirt it comes in contact with will require you to wash it as frequently as if it were your own hair.

It can be difficult to style: If you're not great at styling your own hair, a real hair wig will be just as much work, if not more. It also requires owning a wig stand and a chunk of time to get the job done. Dropping your wig off at a salon to be styled can be pricey.

It gets hot and heavy: If you think about how sweaty and heavy your hair feels in the summer—that's exactly how a real hair wig can feel.

It is expensive: A human-hair wig is basically just a replacement of your own hair—and that comes at a price. The cost of a human hair wig *starts* around £200 and can easily skyrocket up to £2000-plus for top-of-the-line customized wigs.

synthetic hair wigs

While many people associate synthetic wigs with cheap Halloween styles from Party City, the advancement in design, fabrications, and technology means many of them could pass for your own hair. In some cases, it is difficult to tell the difference—the density and texture feel just like human hair.

PROs:

It is easy to maintain: The plastic fibers used to create synthetic hair retain memory, meaning that it maintains its shape no matter what you do to it. If you decide to toss your wig out of a moving car—and then have second thoughts and go back and get it—it will bounce right back into shape. I mean, who doesn't love that?!

No more bad hair days: You know how torturous frizz is on humid days or what a nightmare it is to have to wash and style your strands every time you want to work out? Well, you can kiss that drama goodbye when you have a synthetic wig. "They hold their shape and curl," says Wendy. "So all you have to do is shake it out and plop it on your head and you're good to go."

It is affordable: Synthetic wigs will range from £20 to £200, which affords you the ability to buy a few.

tip: powder your ~~nose~~ hair!

"Synthetic wigs are often very shiny, which can make them look fake," says Wendy Williams. "So, if you put a little baby powder on the wig, then shake it out a bit it will take down the shine a bit. After you shake the baby powder out of the wig, wipe it down with a dry towel" to remove the excess powder.

CONs:

It can't be styled: There are two types of synthetic wigs—regular and heat-resistant. Contrary to its name, heat-resistant synthetic hair should *not* be heat-styled. While a quick blast from the hair dryer or a light once-over with a flat iron is okay, consistent hot heat *will* melt the plastic. With regular synthetic wigs there is no versatility. You can't switch the part, add a curl, or blow-dry it into a style. What you see is what you get.

They don't last: Because they are made from high-performance plastic, synthetic wigs tend to get frayed and knotty with use. Their shelf life is about four to six months.

tip: clean up nicely

Synthetic wigs require specific cleaning and styling products that are geared for fabrics, not hair. Hairspray for synthetic wigs is lighter and will prevent buildup that will make the wig look dirty and feel tacky. To clean a synthetic wig, Wendy advises, "Wash it with Woolite or dish soap in cold water. Then lay it flat to dry. And don't brush it until it's all the way dry. It has memory, all you have to do is shake it."

understanding the *options*

wig construction

Now that you know the two different types of hair options, let's talk about how a wig is created—that is, the construction of it. All the hair has to be attached to something. That something is the cap. There are two types of caps: weft and hand-tied.

Weft wig: The cap is comprised of several vertical pieces of fabric and a series of horizontal wefts—extensionlike sections of hair. The wefts are sewn onto the pieces of fabric by machine. If you turn the wig inside out, it will look like a checkerboard of vertical and horizontal lines of fabric and hair. The downside to a weft wig is that it tends to be heavier because of the interior fabric. Additionally, the part cannot be switched because it will reveal the rows of hair. The upside is that weft wigs are more affordable because they are machine made.

Hand-tied wig: Every single hair is painstakingly hand-crocheted into an ultrathin stocking cap. Imagine a hook rug—that's exactly how these are made. Each strand is individually placed creating the illusion that they are growing out from *your* scalp, allowing versatility with the placement of the part.

base type

Base type describes the type of wig by how it is applied. This is often determined by what is happening with your head in the first place.

Easy On-Off: The name of this type of wig base is self-explanatory. The wig slides on and off the head easily. Those that have temporary hair loss—like us Cancer Cuties—generally use this method of application. They are also the go-to for those with thinning hair and for performers who want or need to wear wigs. Lady Gaga, Cher, Dolly Parton, and the entire cast of *Saturday Night Live*—these are just a few artists who wear easy on-off wigs.

Lace-Front: This type of base is constructed with a lace top–front where the hair is individually hand-tied in order to create a realistic hairline. This is the go-to base for wigs without bangs or for people who want the option of pulling their hair back or wearing updos. Often, this type of wig is glued on in the front so it stays in place for longer durations.

Bonded Wigs: Bonded wigs are those that are glued to the head, just like a man's toupee. They are generally worn by women who have suffered from permanent hair loss caused by medical issues like alopecia. This is generally not recommended for cancer patients because the scalp and skin tend to be sensitive from the chemo and can be irritated by the glue.

wig shopping

Shopping for a wig can be overwhelming especially if you are racing against the chemo clock. Like every other cancer-related appointment, going in educated is key. Follow these tips for ensuring successful shopping and selecting the perfect wig:

book a few consultations

The hospital will supply a list of wig shops. These shops have been vetted for good practices, quality products, educated stylists, and approved by insurance companies. From this list, get referrals from fellow patients or look at reviews online, to narrow down two or three that you will go to for a consultation. Wigs aren't cheap and you want to buy yours from a store that makes you feel comfortable. Wendy also adds, "Avoid the strip mall beauty supply stores. If there are too many green, red, and purple wigs, then that place isn't for you," she says. "Find the boutiques where the Orthodox [Jewish] and black girls go. Ask them, because that's where the best wigs are being made."

do your homework

Before going to your appointment, "do some research," advises Andrew DiSimone, the owner of HairPlaceNYC, a wig salon for cancer patients in New York City. Know the basics so that you can have an educated conversation with the stylist. "Ask questions and don't buy the first wig you see," he adds. Also ask what comes with the cost of the wig. Some shops will "throw in" the cost of the cut or some servicing (the cleaning and styling) at no charge. Booking two, or even three, consultations will allow you to get familiar with what's out there and help you score the best deal.

know your budget

Before you go to your appointment, know your budget. Share this number with the salon staff so that they can help you find a wig that falls within your budget. And don't be embarrassed/afraid/upset if you don't have £2000 to shell out. There are many beautiful wigs that are affordable.

Here's the thing about wig shopping—it's something none of us anticipated we'd have to do. And with it comes unexpected expenses that many of us aren't prepared or equipped to pay for. This is nothing to be ashamed, stressed, or upset about. The good news is there are several organizations that will help you find a quality wig that is both free *and* flattering!

* **National Health Service:** In some cases, wigs are free on the NHS. You can check to see if you qualify here: nhs.uk/NHSEngland/Healthcosts/Pages/wigsandfabricsupports.

* **Friends Are By Your Side:** Celebrity hairstylist Martino Cartier founded this charity to help cancer patients get free wigs through a network of salons across the United States, Canada, Mexico, England, and Australia. Go to www.friendsarebyyourside.com to find a salon in your area.

go while you have hair

Why is this important? If you want to replicate your hair, then it's important for the stylist to see it first. "During the appointment I check out the density of the hair, the formation of the hair, the length, the geometry of your haircut. Is it layered or one length?" says Andrew. "I also check to see what the color is like. Does it have highlights, low lights, or is it one shade?" Basically, it helps a stylist find a perfect match and allows enough time in case one needs to be made.

bring a friend, not an entourage

While it's important to try and have fun when shopping for a wig— it is still an appointment that needs to be taken seriously. Bringing one friend along for moral support is important. Bringing a bunch is bad news. Typically what ends up happening is that your "moral support team" ends up trying on the wigs and you later regret the hooker-blond style you were talked into buying. It's also distracting and overwhelming for the stylist who is trying to help. Andrew warns, "Don't bring your mother or your sister. They love you and will tell you that you look good in everything. Just bring a caring, honest friend who will tell you like it is."

opt for easy

While real-hair wigs are stunning and generally higher quality, there is something to be said for starting with a synthetic wig. "I wouldn't jump into a custom wig if I had never worn wigs before," says Wendy. "Real wigs are a lot of work. My advice is: Keep it simple. Get two or three of the less expensive synthetic ones. They last about a month but maybe by the end of the three-month run your own hair will be growing back."

Andrew weighs in, adding, "I love synthetic, but only when it's not rubbing past your shoulders," he says. "Synthetic is a fiber and when the hair rubs together they fray and get knotty." Keeping the length short (no longer than mid-neck) keeps the wig in good condition. So what do you do if you want longer hair and can't afford a full hand-tied wig? "There are wigs that are a combination of both synthetic and real hair. They have hand-tied tops with real hair and machine-sewn backs where the synthetic hair is." That gives you both the real-looking "scalp" and the long hassle-free length.

mirror your look

While the idea of getting a wig that's drastically different from your own hair might sound exciting, it's probably not the wisest decision when selecting your first wig. There will be days when it's hard to face the bald girl in the mirror. Adding a wig that makes you look even more unrecognizable could make the changes brought on by your cancer harder to deal with. "Stick with your own style and color—or something in that family—until you are comfortable wearing a wig," advises Wendy. "I was only comfortable playing after wearing wigs for several years. Give yourself a moment to adjust."

tip: keep it real!

Bangs, baby hairs, and visible roots are little details that make a wig look like a real head of hair, Wendy says. If you find a wig that you love but feel the color is one-dimensional, bring it to your colorist and have them darken the roots. If it's a synthetic wig, a little brown mascara or shadow applied along the part can mimic a natural root line.

wig *accessories* that will make your life *easier*

Wearing wigs can be—to put it mildly—uncomfortable. Almost every cancer patient I know or interviewed shared how itchy and hot their heads were when wearing their wigs, how high-maintenance they are, and how tricky it can be to style them. While these facts are relatively inescapable there are a few beauty products and gadgets that can make your life easier. Joan Lunden dishes about the key accessories that will make wearing your wig more comfortable and easier to maintain. Below are her wig-wearing essentials:

wig chin styling strap

It can be frustrating—and tricky—to try and style a wig that won't sit still on your head. "One thing that I found very helpful was a wig chin styling strap," says Joan. "It is an elastic cord with alligator clamps on both ends. You clip one clamp to one side of the wig, then wrap the little cord under your chin, and then clip the other clamp to the other side of the wig. It helps keep your wig in place so you can use a blow-dryer with a round brush to finish off the styling while it's on your head."

Try: www.headcovers.com

wig stand

"I am always on the go—making speeches and appearances and I would bring the portable plastic stand with me," says Joan. "I can take them apart and the pieces lie flat in my suitcase. But they are great because if the wig is warm or damp on the inside, it allows the air to circulate and dry the inside. When you put a wig on, you want it to be dry."

Styrofoam stands tend to be larger than real heads and can stretch out your wig. To prevent that, try this beauty hack: Use a measuring tape to figure out the size of your head. Then, measure the Styrofoam to figure out the difference in size. To make sure it replicates the size of your noggin, use a serrated knife to cut off the discrepancy from the back of the form head. Finish by wrapping the form with duct tape to prevent any Styrofoam bits from breaking off and getting in your wig.

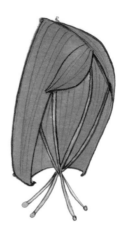

Try: www.wowwigs.com

wig caps

Wig grips, caps, and liners are disposable head covers made from thin high-tech fabrics that provide a protective barrier between the scalp and the wig. They help wick sweat from the head, allow the skin to breathe and minimize itchiness. "They are great because when you put them on, the inside of the wig doesn't touch your head and that's what makes your head itch," shares Joan. These are essential if you need or plan to wear a wig every day. So, let's talk about the different functions of liners, caps, and grips so you know what will work best for you.

Wig liners come in two basic styles:

Nylon liners look exactly like pantyhose and provide the scalp with a soft, smooth layer of protection from the rubbing, irritation, or heat caused by the wig. They are best for those without hair.

Mesh liners look like fishnet stockings and are used primarily to help prevent the wig from slipping or moving around. The netted holes allow for them to be used with wig clips and combs, which help secure the wig to existing hair. "This looser weave is not quite as hot" as the nylon liners, adds Joan.

Try: www.voguewigs.com

tip: put a cap on it!

Since wig liners are delicate just like stockings, they tend to rip or tear easily. Buy some that are sold in multipacks so you have backups available if/when your caps rip. Also, when putting on a wig cap, make sure to put it on from the nape of your neck first stretching it upward until it reaches and covers up to your forehead and hairline. Doing it this way makes it easier to adjust and keeps it from slipping back on the head.

wig grips

Wig grips look like a wide headband and cover only a small section of the head. Generally, these bands are constructed with textured fabric and an adjustable closure. They can be wrapped and positioned anywhere on the head—along the hairline or farther back—to help keep scarves or wigs firmly in place. My favorite is The Hair Grip. This band is made from velour and grips to both the scalp and wigs. Its hold is so strong that it nixes the need for clips and combs. Wanna whip your hair back and forth? Then get a grip!

Try: www.thehairgrip.com

halo hair

"I got these things that were like a half wig," says Joan. "It has a circular band that goes around your head and sits right on your forehead. Hair extensions are attached to a band and hang down like regular hair. They come with bangs, some without." Halo hair pieces are great for wearing under hats or a bandana when you don't want to wear a full wig for whatever reason. "When you have a hat or bandana over it, nobody would ever know that you are bald. To me, it made me feel like I looked like me. And when I looked like me, I felt better about myself and I felt stronger," she says. "I know it's psychological but there's something to be said for the importance of the psychological when you are battling cancer."

Try: www.headcovers.com

done with treatment? don't toss your wig—donate it!

Done with treatment and wondering what you should do with your second set of locks? The answer is simple: Donate it! There are many woman and young girls now walking in your shoes—so why shouldn't they wear your hair as well! If you have a wig stored away or collecting dust on its wig stand, this is a great opportunity to help out another cancer patient. Below are some places that participate in wig donations programs. You will need to call to find one that will take yours. Don't delay—do it today!

* **Cancer centers:** Ring the cancer center where you had treatment and ask if they donate wigs to patients. If they don't, they will know who does.

* **Wig shops:** Most wig shops make a habit of donating a certain amount of wigs to patients who don't have the resources to purchase a new one. Shops that don't have a donation program will be in the know on local wig drives and can inform you of dates and times you can drop off yours.

* **Cancer Research UK or Macmillan:** There are local chapters that may provide free wigs to cancer patients and places where you can drop off your wig for donation.

cold cap *therapy:* keeping your hair during chemo

For many women, keeping their hair during treatment is a priority. For some, it's about privacy in the workplace. For others, it's about maintaining a sense of self. For others still, it's about protecting their children from knowing a horrible truth. Whatever the reason, cold cap therapy, a treatment that can help you keep or preserve your hair during chemo treatment, is gaining popularity. In December 2015 the Food and Drug Administration cleared the first scalp-cooling device, the DigniCap. There are three other companies in the United States that also offer cold cap therapy: Penguin Cold Caps, Chemo Cold Caps, and Arctic Cold Caps.

This hair-saving treatment uses snug, gel-filled hats, chilled to −15 to −45 degrees Fahrenheit, to help constrict the blood vessels, limiting the amount of chemotherapy that reaches the scalp. It is also believed that the cold temps help reduce the metabolic activity of the follicular cells, reducing the effectiveness of the chemo on the hair.

The caps, which vary in design from company to company, resemble a combination of an ice pack and a swim cap. They are worn for hours before, during, and after each chemotherapy treatment. In order to maintain a consistent, cold temperature, four caps are stored in a portable medical cooler over dry ice and patients are required to rotate caps every twenty to thirty minutes.

Be warned: This treatment isn't comfortable. "It's really cold and I would get a bad freezer burn headache that lasted for the first two caps," says Torva Durkin, forty-four, who opted to do the therapy when she was diagnosed with breast cancer. "It was so cold there would be ice chips in my hair." To keep warm while wearing a sub-zero cap, patients bundle up in electric blankets, layers of socks, and even wear moleskin or panty liners on their forehead and around their ears for protection.

Cold cap therapy is also a big time commitment. "I don't think people realize how much work it is and the time commitment it requires," she adds. "There were days I would be in the chemo room for twelve or thirteen hours. You have to have the cap on for fifty minutes before chemo, then you have the infusion, which takes four and a half hours, and then you have to wear the caps for four and a half hours post-infusion." Patients can hire trained "cappers" who will tote the coolers and ensure the rotation and application of the caps is done properly and efficiently. Some hospitals don't have facilities for scalp cooling. Your doctor or chemotherapy nurse can tell you if it's available and if it's suitable for you.

If you are considering or about to start cold cap therapy, below are some tips that will help you hold on to your hair.

tips for cold cap therapy

1 Opt for shampoo that has a similar pH to that of the hair—in the 4.5 to 5.5 range. An easy way to find a shampoo with those pH levels are ones labeled "gentle."

2 Normally, "moisturizing" and "volumizing" shampoos are great for the hair but when you are doing cold cap therapy, they can actually coat the hair and keep oxygen from reaching the follicles. One way to know these shampoos by sight is that they appear "milky" or "creamy." Instead, choose shampoos that are clear. Most cold cap companies have specific hair care brands they will recommend you use during therapy. Once you get that list, start using those products immediately as it can take up to two weeks or more for residue of old products to get off the hair. Instead of using heavy conditioners, Torva suggests using a detangling spray or leave-in conditioner. It provides necessary moisture to the hair without coating the follicles. Again, each cold cap company will provide their specific product recommendations.

3 Coloring hair is not recommended until three months after chemo is finished, because the follicles still need time to recover from the trauma of chemotherapy. If your roots start to show before you can get to the salon, Torva suggests her go-to: "The Color Wow Root Cover Up is easy to brush on and is the best at hiding any grays," she said (www.colorwowhair.com).

4 Avoiding friction on the hair will help avoid pressure and pulling on the follicle. Sleeping on a satin pillowcase may sound like a diva move but it will save your strands while you snooze.

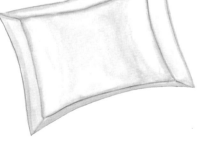

5 This is a rule for anyone having chemotherapy but even more important to follow for those who are doing cold cap therapy: Do NOT, I repeat,

DO NOT use heat tools. They stress strands and follicles and lead to hair loss. This includes curling irons, flat irons, and hair dryers.

6 Cold caps are called "cold caps" for a reason; they are super cold. So cold they can cause freezer burn and blisters. When wearing the caps, Torva would use maxi pads as a protective barrier to shield her forehead. Another option is adhesive-backed moleskin, which is thinner but also does the job. Opt for a padding roll of Moleskin Plus by Dr. Scholl's, which can be custom cut for whatever size area you want or need to cover.

7 The upside to cold cap therapy is you keep a lot of your hair. The downside is that it does thin out quite a bit. To help camouflage this hair loss, fiber-based powders (similar to dry shampoos) work wonders to conceal patchy or thin spots. My top picks are Nanogen Keratin Hair Fibers (www.nanogenhair.com), Toppik Hair Building Fibers (toppik.com), and Viviscal Conceal & Densify Volumizing Fibers (www.viviscal.com). If you are considering cold cap therapy, a great source of information can be found on the Macmillan website or at the Rapunzel Project (www.rapunzelproject.org). I highly suggest that you check out these websites before beginning treatment.

tip: nix hair dramas in a snap!

During cold cap therapy hair thins and cannot be colored. "I came up with a fix for both problems," says Torva. "I purchased clip-in Remy human hair extensions on eBay in a few colors to match my highlighted hair. The great thing about these extensions is that you can curl them with an iron. I also purchased a bunch of small infinity scarves and cotton headbands from Forever 21, Walgreens, and Kohl's for about two or three dollars each. I take the extensions and snap them onto the edge of headbands, then slip it onto my head. Voilà—I have a full head of hair and my grays are covered!"

While cold cap therapy has been a regular part of cancer treatment in Europe for almost twenty years, it is important to note that there is a percentage of the American medical community that remains concerned that the caps may prevent chemotherapy from reaching the scalp—leaving behind potential cancerous cells that could be lurking there. Studies conducted in Germany show that the use of cold caps does not increase the risk of skin metastases. However, more studies are needed to conclusively determine its safety and efficacy. Talk to your doctor to weigh the pros and cons and then decide what course of treatment benefits your health and your quality of life the most.

hair-raising: posttreatment *strands*

Each type of therapy—chemo, cold cap, and radiation—will have an effect on your hair. It is well documented that women who undergo chemotherapy experience a change in their texture and curl pattern, dubbed "chemo curls." For those who had cold cap therapy or CMF chemotherapy where hair thinning is the name of the game, strands can grow back with a kinky bend or stick straight. For those who had radiation, strands will be zapped of moisture and shine. There is no science behind why these changes occur. Most scientists and hairstylists point to cellular changes in the follicle. But the important takeaway is that it's all temporary. And the upside is that you may just find a new style that looks even better on you. That's exactly what happened to Joan. After years of wearing a preppy blond bob, she ended up with an even more sophisticated crop. "If my hairdresser ever would have said to me, 'Let's cut your hair short, like a quarter of an inch on both sides,' I would have said, 'What, are you on drugs?' I never would have done it," she says. "Now, I think I have an even better style and it takes me less than forty-five minutes!"

what you need to know about your post-cancer hair

anticipate changes

Chemo and radiation linger in your body for six months to a year. This will be reflected in your hair, skin, and nails. Not only will your hair texture change but it will react to products differently as well. This includes salon treatments like coloring and straightening treatments. "When my hair started growing back, I said to my colorist, 'Just make me blond again.' I know there's only a quarter of an inch there but if I'm going to look like a Chia Pet, then I want to be a blond Chia Pet," says Joan. After her colorist dyed her hair, the blond quickly oxidized to a bright shade of orange. "The next weekend, I was at some Race for the Cure in the Survivors' Tent and someone said to me, 'Oh, by the way, when you color your hair for the first time after treatment, it turns bright orange or green.

It has something to do with the chemicals still in your system.' You can't expect everything to go back to normal right away. It just doesn't." The key here is to wait as long as you can before coloring or processing your hair. If you can wait—ideally, six months—you stand to look prettier for it.

switch up your products

Most likely, the products you used on your hair before—shampoos to styling products—won't work on your post-chemo hair the same way they did before. You will need moisturizing cleansers and conditioners to up your hair's hydration and stronger styling products to tame the unruly curls. I dipped into my boyfriend's stash of pomade and gel—and that seemed to do the trick. The point being: You are going to have to whip up some hair cocktails and experiment to see what works now. My advice, don't get frustrated. Have fun with it. You have hair again after all—so try to keep a positive perspective.

mini tools deliver big

When your hair is less than two inches, a paddle brush is basically worthless. Investing in smaller mini tools will allow you to make your short strands stylish. My favorite mini round brush, the Ibiza EX1, is only one and half inches and has nylon and boar bristles, perfect for styling pompadours and pixies. It's also amazing for taming short frizz and flyaways along the root line (www.ibizahair.com). An itty-bitty flat iron will also help smooth curls to help you achieve a more polished look. Brands such as ghd, T3, CHI, and Babyliss offer mini irons that won't damage your hair. When hair is through the transitional phases, keep these tools handy and use them when traveling.

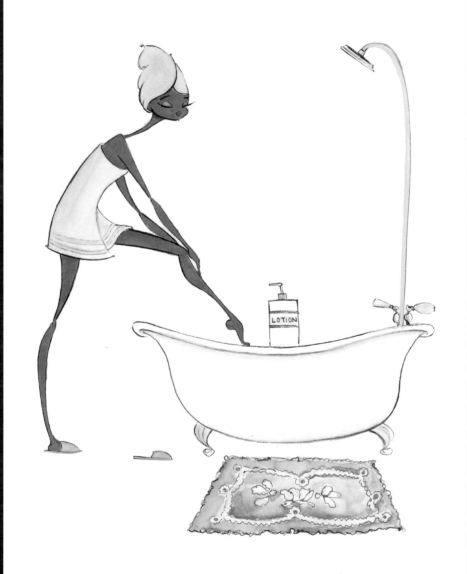

CHAPTER 3

BEAUTY *IS* SKIN DEEP

how to care for the skin you're in

Skin. It's the largest—and heaviest—organ of our body. It can measure more than five feet long and weigh up to eight pounds! While most of us focus on the visual condition of our skin, we often forget how critical it is to our survival. Our skin is basically a fleshy coat of armor. It shields our tissues, blood vessels, and internal organs against bacteria, extreme temperatures, and damaging sunlight—it even protects us from physical harm when we fall or get cut. But it does *soooo* much more than that. The skin contains a massive network of nerve endings and touch receptors that fire signals to the brain alerting us to potential dangers—and pleasures—we come in contact with. The tip of the finger alone contains approximately 2,500 nerve receptors. And you wonder why a paper cut hurts so badly…

what's happening *internally* affects you *externally*

The good news:

Lizards, worms, and starfish aren't the only creatures that can regenerate parts of their bodies. Humans can too! While we may not be as adept at it as these little critters, our skin has an amazing ability to grow back and repair itself. The upper layers of the skin are made up of rapidly dividing cells that undergo a full regeneration cycle every twenty-seven days, giving it the power to heal itself when it gets cut, burned, or harmed. Those cells are found in the epidermis (the surface layer of our skin), in our scalp and hair follicles, in the matrix of our nails, even in the mucous membranes of the mouth and nose. These cells are the reason our hair and nails grow, our skin glows—and basically—why we look so fabulous. (And yes, we do!)

The bad news:

Most chemotherapies, even some of the new immunotherapies, are targeted to wipe out and destroy rapidly dividing cancer cells. Problem is, since these chemicals can't determine cancer cells from healthy cells—the treatment kills ALL rapidly dividing cells in the body. That means our skin, hair, and nails take a direct hit. Hair falls out. Skin gets itchy, dry, and irritated. Nails become brittle, peel, and break. Like it's not enough that we feel like crap—now we have to look like it, too? While some side effects are inevitable, there are easy things we can do to keep our skin healthy and in good condition. (Holla for those silver linings!)

skin care *during* treatment

"Baby aspirin can cause bruising," says Dr. Donald F. Richey, a board-certified dermatologist and founder of Brighter Days, a California-based program that helps cancer patients deal with skin-related side effects of chemotherapy and radiation. "So you can just imagine what a toxic chemical can do to your body."

He makes a good point.

The side effects of chemo and radiation are long and varied: dry skin, rashes, flushing, acnelike breakouts, itching, peeling, photosensitivity, blisters, hives, scaly patches, becoming retro-dermic (red from head to toe)—and the list goes on and on. Reactions vary from person to person and are based on the type of chemotherapy you receive, the condition your skin was in before you began treatment, and how sensitive your skin is.

I don't know why, but I was shocked by how jacked my skin got. In many ways, I was still grappling with the reality that I had breast cancer. It was the side effects that actually forced me to acknowledge I was sick. "Denial ain't just a river in Egypt…"

"All of a sudden, around day fourteen, your oil glands shut down and you become dry, very dry and with that's when you get skin rashes, infections, et cetera," says Dr. Richey. "But the biggest thing is dry skin."

If by dry skin he means resembling an armadillo girdled lizard, then yeah, that's about right. (Google it, to see what I mean.) By my third treatment, my skin became so dry it started to shed and where I wasn't shedding I had red, sore hivelike bumps. It didn't get better as time went on. On the days after my chemo I would turn a sickly shade of pus green. It was NOT a good look. But I'm not a girl who settles for anything less than being fabulous—so I turned to my squad of dermatologists to figure out how to turn this ugly situation around. This is the advice I got….

time to rethink your routine

Let me guess how your beauty routine goes down each morning: You wake up, jump in a long, hot shower, exfoliate your body, shave your pits and legs, and suds up until you're squeaky clean. After you get out, it's a rough 'n' tumble towel off, before finishing with a fragrant body lotion. Am I right?

That is exactly what I used to do. But as you know by now, cancer changes things—and you need to adjust your routine if you want to look and feel your best. Here's why: The body has a love-hate relationship with water. Internally, it is key for keeping our organs, muscles, and tissues hydrated and healthy. Externally, it can be one of the harshest elements for our body to endure. Crazy, right? Too much water on the skin, hair, and nails actually has the opposite effect you would think—zapping it of necessary moisture. Drinking plenty of water is essential throughout our lives but it becomes critical when we have harmful toxins rushing through our veins. At the same time, patients need to be careful how much water they are exposing their bodies to. Stressing out an already weak system is, as I like to say, "no bueno."

"Don't fall into the trap of over-cleansing, over-scrubbing, and overusing everything antibacterial in order to prevent a secondary infection," says Dr. Heidi Waldorf, director of Laser and Cosmetic

tip: don't get the slip!

Before stepping foot into a bath or shower, make sure you have a good mat with a rubber bottom to prevent you from slipping. When you're in chemo and not feeling your best, you might not be the steadiest on your feet. A bath mat made from memory foam provides a grip for your tootsies and (just in case you fall) a cushion for your tushie.

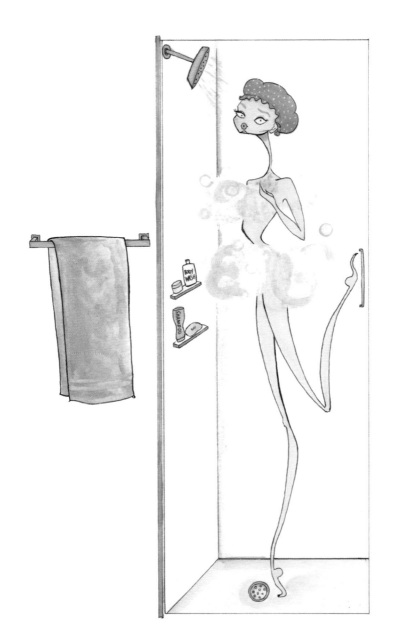

Dermatology at the Icahn School of Medicine at Mount Sinai in New York City and founder of Waldorf Dermatology & Laser Associates in Nanuet, New York. She is also a survivor of stage IIB invasive ductal carcinoma breast cancer. "If you strip the skin, it's going to be more open and more prone to outside environmental issues."

limit your shower to ten minutes (or less)

If you are anything like me, you love a long, steamy shower. Whenever I am stressed, depressed, or just wiped out, nothing feels better than warm water beating down on my body. It seems to wash all my troubles away while soothing my sore, tired muscles. Sadly, this is an indulgence you will have to put on hold for now.

Water strips the skin of its natural oils, leaving it exposed and prone to irritation. Instead, keep your shower or bath short—ten minutes, tops. As for the temperature of the water—keep it tepid or warm. If your bathroom starts to steam up, it's a sign that the water is too hot. If I were you, I'd skip a bath altogether. Sitting in stagnant water with dirt, oil, and germs floating around in it is unhygienic. If you have even the tiniest cut, it can lead to an infection. A shower is the most effective way to get all the funk from your body down the drain. But whatever your preference, bath or shower, just make sure you don't dillydally.

tip: be a clock-watcher

Do you linger in the bath or shower *waaaay* too long? If so, use your kitchen timer as an easy way to clock your minutes under the water. Trust me, it's a serious skin-saver. Turn the dial to ten. When the buzzer sounds—it's time to hop out and towel off.

opt for a pima pat-down

Rubbing a towel over your wet body seems an efficient way to get dry fast—and it is. But it's also rough on the skin. Instead, patting down with a soft towel will help you dry off without drying up. Towels made from Egyptian cotton are the most absorbent, making them a popular pick. However, towels made from Peruvian cotton are the best for those with sensitive skin. Peruvian pima grows in the rich soil located along the coast of the country, making it the softest and smoothest. Bonus: The cotton fibers are also very long, so it's less likely to shed or produce lint. Score!

moisturize, moisturize, moisturize

After you finish patting down, when skin is still a little damp, slather yourself in a rich body lotion, cream, or oil to seal in moisture. As you rub it into your skin, take the time to enjoy the process of pampering yourself. I would use these few private moments in the bathroom to set my intentions for the day, express my gratitude to the powers that be, and to get in the right frame of mind to face the day. It's a ritual I continue today and it's truly cathartic.

"My body lotions and oils are things that make me feel the happiest and calmest in the morning and at night," says Sandra Lee, the Emmy-winning lifestyle expert, chef, author, and TV host. Sandra is also a DCIS, stage 0 breast cancer survivor.

"Throughout this process, I have used ESPA Soothing Body Oil. It is an aromatic blend that destresses the body and mind. It hydrates my skin and the smell is so calming."

tip: sleep on this!

"Get a humidifier for your bedroom to make sure you are getting enough moisture in the room where you sleep," advises Dr. Doris Day, New York City–based dermatologist, medical journalist, clinical associate professor of dermatology at NYU, and author of the book *Forget the Facelift*. Doing this in the p.m. ensures you wake up with hydrated, glowing skin in the a.m. "You want to do it until it almost fogs up the windows."

skin care: organic versus nonorganic

The minute I was diagnosed, I read everything I could get my hands on about caring for my body during this journey. For each new phase of treatment, I would research and read all I could. I wanted to be ready for what was about to happen to me and be prepared to deal with it. One of the things I read time and time again was that organic products are safer for cancer patients to use than traditional or well-known skin care lines. I find this almost offensive. This is information that is NOT based in science and preys on the fears of those facing the most harrowing time of their lives. I have interviewed some of the top dermatologists in the United States for this book and they all agree on this point. So, let's set the record straight right now.

"The whole all-organic thing is nonsense because there is no standard for organics in skin care. There is in food but not in skin care," says Dr. Day. "I like to remind my patients that poison ivy is natural but you don't go rubbing that all over your skin. Arsenic, mercury, and lead are also natural ingredients. Organic products tend to have a higher incidence of containing them."

The point being: organic versus nonorganic isn't so black and white. Don't get me wrong, I love products that are well formulated and pure—but sometimes "organic" products aren't the best for those with heightened skin issues. For example, coconut oil is all the rage right now and while it's great for a multitude of beauty treatments—conditioning the hair, removing makeup, et cetera—it's not the most effective moisturizer cancer patients can use.

"There is nothing special about coconut oil," says Dr. Waldorf. "You are better off moisturizing with a good therapeutic cream. Most oils, including coconut oil, are occlusive. It doesn't contain any humectants for holding more moisture or any emollients to make the skin silky. It's just not the best choice."

Ingredients are one thing, but the delivery systems are just as important. How amazing is coconut oil—or any ingredient for that matter—if it can't penetrate into the layers of the skin? The answer: not so great. So, before you write off any mainstream products because they aren't organic, you might want to consider the technologies of the formulas first. Case in point: Back in the day, our grandparents and parents would sit in a bath filled with oatmeal to help soothe their irritated skin. Today, brands like Aveeno have the technology to isolate the part of the oat that alleviates irritations and formulate it with moisturizing ingredients. The result is that the oat becomes more effective because it can be absorbed faster and deeper into the dermis. Personally, I prefer to rely on products that are science- and evidence-backed. Plus, who the hell wants to clean soggy, sticky oatmeal out of their tub? Not me.

Since understanding ingredient lists on skin care products can be harder than reading hieroglyphics, I asked Karen Hohenstein, cosmetic chemist who has formulated beauty products for brands including Neutrogena, Redken, and Alterna, to come to our rescue.

"You may have some unwelcome changes during treatment but choosing the right products can help you feel comfortable in your own skin," says Karen. "The ideal products are gentle and mild, nondrying, hypoallergenic, and free of irritating dyes, fragrances, and preservatives." Below is her easy-to-understand breakdown of ingredients to look for and how they help.

the power players—ingredients to look for

emollients

How they help: These ingredients add smoothness to rough, dry skin and help hold in moisture.

What to look for: Natural shea and cocoa butters have a rich, velvety texture. Oils such as olive and sunflower spread easily and have a soft, smooth feel. Fatty acids such as stearic acid help rebuild the skin's cell membrane and natural moisture barrier function. Dimethicone, a silicone-based emollient, forms a protective barrier against irritants. Don't be deterred by names like cetyl and stearyl alcohols—they are *not* drying alcohols but actually waxy emollients that help bind moisture into the skin.

humectants

How they help: These water-soluble compounds bind moisture into the skin. If you think about how a sponge looks when it's dry and how it instantly expands after it comes into contact with water—that's exactly how humectants work in the skin. For example, hyaluronic acid holds up to a thousand times its weight in water and leaves skin looking plump and youthful.

What to look for: glycerin, hyaluronic acid or sodium hyaluronate, sodium PCA, sodium lactate, amino acids, and panthenol.

anti-irritants

How they help: These ingredients are used to soothe and calm rough, irritated skin. They help increase the water content of the skin cells, enhance cell turnover and proliferation, and speed up wound healing.

What to look for: allantoin, calendula extract, and oatmeal.

ceramides/ceramide analogs

How they work: Ceramides are lipids (fats) that form a layered structure, like a stack of pancakes, which reinforces the natural lipid barrier of the skin. The ceramide layers hold water in the dermis, keeping it moisturized. In recent trials on people with xerosis (pathologically dry skin), moisturizers formulated with ceramides outperformed other moisturizers by actually repairing the structure of the skin and improving its ability to maintain its own moisture balance. Ceramides are expensive so some companies use cheaper materials that mimic them. These are called "ceramide analogs palmitamides." Phospholipids and sphingolipids are similar, usually used in combination with cholesterol.

What to look for: Ceramides are listed by number: ceramide-1, ceramide-3, ceramide 6-11, et cetera. Palmitamides are listed as cetyl-PG hydroxyethyl palmitamide. Phospholipids and sphingolipids will be listed as phytosphingosine or lecithin.

peptides

How they work: These materials are the result of the latest research into skin function. Peptides stimulate the production of collagen and other structural fibers, increasing density and resilience of skin.

What to look for: palmitoyl tetrapeptide-3 and myristoyl tripeptide-31.

suggested skin care products

facial cleanser and body wash

The intel: Typical cleansers and body washes are formulated with sulfate-based surfactants, which may be too drying and irritating for sensitive skin. Look for ones that are sulfate-free. Or opt for ultra-mild baby wash products that perform well as a facial cleanser or body wash, and can even double as a gentle shampoo.

Some suggestions: CeraVe Hydrating Cleanser, Cetaphil Gentle Skin Cleanser, Cetaphil RestoraDerm Eczema Calming Body Wash, Cetaphil Cleansing Bar, Dove Sensitive Skin Body Wash with Nutri-umMoisture, Dove Sensitive Skin Body Bar, Johnson's Baby Naturals Head-to-Toe Wash, CeraVe Baby Wash & Shampoo, Burt's Bees Baby Bee Shampoo & Wash, Tom's of Maine Baby Shampoo & Wash, and Baby Hugo Naturals Shampoo & Baby Wash.

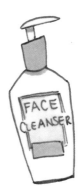

body cream and lotion

The Intel: A body cream or lotion packed with emollients, humectants, and peptides will hydrate and replenish the skin. If you are experiencing any irritations like rashes, itching, or dry patches, opt for creams that are formulated for anti-itch or eczema treatment—they'll give you the most relief.

Some suggestions: CeraVe Moisturizing Cream or Lotion; Avène Professional TriXera + Selectiose Emollient Cream; Aveeno Active Naturals Skin Relief Moisture Repair Cream; Aveeno Anti-Itch Concentrated Lotion; Aveeno Active Naturals Eczema Therapy Moisturizing Cream; Caudalie Vine Body Butter; Cetaphil RestoraDerm Eczema Calming Body Moisturizer; Curél Itch Defense Lotion; and

Eucerin Eczema Relief Body Creme, all enriched with ceramides and calming ingredients. If all else fails, try super-gentle baby lotions, such as Aveeno Baby Eczema Therapy Moisturizing Cream, CeraVe Baby Moisturizing Cream, and Eucerin Eczema Relief Baby Lotion.

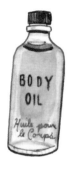

body oil

The Intel: Your skin may be so dry that even the extra-moisturizing versions of body creams and lotions won't do the trick. Using them in tandem with a body oil, which helps rebuild and protect the hydrolipidic film of the dermis, will help restore your skin to its former glory. Opt for unscented or lightly scented versions, which are gentler.

Some suggestions: My favorite oils are Avène Body Oil, Neutrogena Body Oil, Rodin Olio Lusso Body Oil, and Indie Lee Moisturizing Oil. No matter how many custom-blended or prestige body oils I got to test as a beauty director, I would always go back to one of these. The Rodin is expensive, so it was my splurge during chemo. Every time I used it, I felt seriously pampered. But all four—in my opinion—feel equally luxurious. After showering, towel off, then pour a quarter-sized amount of the oil into your palm and massage into your legs. Repeat for the entire body. Then apply body lotion, which will trap in the moisture and help eliminate any greasy feel.

facial moisturizer

The Intel: Many "daytime" facial moisturizers contain SPF, and, for the most part, I am totally on board for anything that makes my life easier. Eliminate one step from my morning routine and I'm already a happier woman. I'm sure you feel the same way. *But*—and this is a big *but*—moisturizers with SPF generally don't contain adequate levels of sun

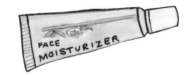

protection for those undergoing chemotherapy. Plus, SPF—when applied directly to skin, without a layer of moisturizer to create a protective barrier—can be irritating. Opt for moisturizers without SPF or just use your "nighttime" or "p.m." version during the day as well.

Some suggestions: CeraVe Facial Moisturizing Lotion PM, Olay Active Hydrating Beauty Fluid Lotion, and the cult-classic Embryolisse Lait Cream Concentrate are three that get my thumbs-up.

face masks

The Intel: Every once in a while we need a little extra somethin' somethin' to make us look and feel our best. For me, this hero helper is a face mask. Personally, I am obsessed with Korean sheet masks with their easy application and unique ingredients (snail or donkey

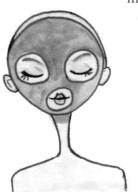

milk anyone?). I slap one on and then catch up on the TV shows I missed during the week. Regardless of the type of mask you prefer, they work wonders to refresh and refine the skin.

Some suggestions: Sheet masks from Karuna and It's Skin are amazing. "I use Fango Active Mud Mask for Face and Body by Borghese," says Sandra of her mineral-rich pick. "I put it on and ten minutes later my skin is just glowing. It's really incredible."

sunscreen

The Intel: You are wearing sunscreen every day, right? You better be! Chemotherapy increases sun sensitivity and even subtle exposure to the sun's harmful UVA and UVB rays can leave unsightly sunspots faster than it normally takes. "I got a few freckles from the short walks home after work," says Dr. Waldorf. "Once I realized this was

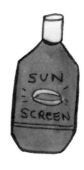

happening, at the end of the day I would throw my wig in a ziplock bag and put on a large, wide-brimmed hat. I would reapply my sunblock—and not just on my face—but on back of my neck, my hands, and any part of my skin that was exposed." Traditional chemical sunscreens that contain homosalate, octocrylene, avobenzone, et cetera, can be irritating so opt for mineral sunscreens with titanium dioxide and zinc oxide. They are just as effective and protective but way more gentle.

Some suggestions: Colorescience Sunforgettable Mineral Sunscreen, La Roche-Posay Anthelios 50 Mineral Ultra Light Sunscreen Fluid, Hang Ten Mineral Sport Sunscreen SPF 30. Two of my favorites are: Neutrogena Pure & Free Baby Sunscreen SPF 60+—the whiteness disappears within seconds and the nongreasy product works well under makeup; and Neutrogena Ultra Sheer Liquid Daily Sunscreen Broad Spectrum 70, which gives my skin a dewy glow.

lip balm

The Intel: There are certain body parts that show warning signs when something is wrong with our health. Nails are one. Lips are another. The mouth is also one of the few parts of the body that does not contain oil glands. The upside is that the minute you start to experience a vitamin deficiency or dehydration, your lips will let you know. The downside is that they require extra love and attention to keep them in good condition. Look for balms formulated with beeswax, oils (olive and jojoba), vitamin E, hyaluronic acid, honey, propolis, and shea butter.

Some suggestions: My top picks include: Burt's Bees Ultra Conditioning Lip Balm with Kokum Butter, Avène Cold Cream Lip Balm, Beessential Honey Lip Balm, Nuxe Rêve de Miel Ultra-Nourishing Lip Balm, EOS Lip Balm, Fresh Sugar Lip Treatment.

Steer clear of ingredients that are drying like petroleum jelly and minty flavors made with menthol or eucalyptus. Also avoid balms that are packaged in pots and tubs. The last thing you want to do is transfer nasty germs from your fingertips to your mouth. Stick tubes are the most sanitary.

tip: seal it with a kiss

There can be a benefit to off-label repurposing...Whenever my pout feels dry or sore and I have no lip balm hanging around, I reach for a few products that aren't necessarily made to heal the lips, but do so anyway. Dior Creme Abricot is a cuticle cream that transforms my nails but its sweet, waxy balm also makes my lips soft and supple. I also love the Australian cult classic, Lucas' Papaw Ointment, and the French version, Homeoplasmine. Both look and feel like they have a petroleum base but they are actually fruit- and plant-derived balms that are nothing short of miracle workers. Plus, they can be used all over the body—so it's a beauty bargain to boot!

putting your best face forward with retinol, antioxidants, and botox?

There are some of you who will experience very mild reactions or none at all during treatment. Lucky ladies! Because of this, you might want to pick up where you left off with your regular beauty routine. That might include using retinols, antioxidants, even fillers like Botox and Restylane. Before you do, you need to get the thumbs-up from your oncologist. Most oncologists don't want their patients eating, drinking, or applying anything that can affect your treatment—and some of these ingredients and products can and will.

Let me tell you why.

There is a phenomenon called radiation recall dermatitis (RRD) and chemotherapy recall dermatitis (CRD) where chemotherapy drugs, or even certain strong skin care ingredients, can induce an inflammatory reaction at a previous injury site. So, let's say you had a bad burn on your hand years ago: Some chemotherapies or even strong creams used during chemo can make it reappear.

RRD (or CRD) most often displays itself in the skin but can also affect the organs including the lungs, esophagus, intestinal epithelium, oral mucosa, bladder mucosa, and heart. "Even if you're not being treated in one particular area, when you're going through chemotherapy using retinoic acid may be too harsh and could cause a flare-up," says Dr. Day. "Retinol can also increase your risk of infection if your skin is not intact." The good news is there is a nice alternative. "During treatment I would do pro-retinols, the over-the-counter version, that are more gentle because they're not prescription. Roc, Olay, and Neutrogena have good pro-retinols that are gentle but effective."

Oncologists also have equal concerns regarding antioxidants. "But wait!" you say. "Aren't antioxidants good for me?" Normally, yes. The most popular ones, vitamin C, E, and A, are formulated into our serums, eye treatments, and face creams because of their abilities to boost collagen production, prevent the oxidation of our skin, and minimize sun and age spots. There are also plant-derived antioxidants called phytonutrients. The most well known of these are beta-carotene (found in carrots), lycopene (from beans, like chickpeas), and my favorite—resveratrol (from wine!!!!). These molecules safeguard our cells from oxidation. Image a bank robbery in progress: The robbers are the free radicals that cause skin cells to oxidize and wither. The antioxidants are the police officers that arrive on the scene to bust up the robbery and save our skin. Antioxidants are skin care heroes.

However, during treatment, these cell-saving molecules aren't such a good thing.

"People are all about antioxidants," says Dr. Waldorf. "But antioxidants can limit the damage your chemo is doing to the cancer cells." In other words, antioxidants help keep cancer cells alive. My oncologist put the kibosh on using any antioxidants. I was even surprised when he told me to stop taking my oral supplements and juicing. But I followed his orders because I wanted to make sure my chemo was as effective as it could be. My thought is, why risk it? In only a matter of months you'll be able to take or use whatever you want again.

As for injectables including Botox and Restylane—most oncologists aren't going to sign off on you putting toxins and unnatural chemicals in your body. That's sorta a no-brainer. However, by the time you are wrapping up treatment, your face might appear hallow and gaunt. This is where injectables can help provide a visual—and, often times, emotional—pick-me-up.

Now, I know what you're thinking: "You're telling me to get Botox while I have cancer?!" Hear me out.

First, I am not telling you to do anything. And you should *always, always, always* check with your doctor before doing *any* cosmetic treatment. That said, there have been no studies—NONE—that link Botox, Restylane, or any other injectable to causing or fueling cancer. If there were, the FDA would not approve them for use. In many ways, this is similar to the organic versus nonorganic argument because both are fueled by emotion and not rooted in scientific evidence. I have been on both sides of this argument—as a beauty director and a cancer patient—and I make my decisions as a patient based on the medical evidence and the studies.

What most people don't know is that in 2006, *Clinical Cancer Research* published a study revealing that Botox, used as an adjuvant treatment, could actually help target resistant tumors.

Additional recent studies have yielded similar results. While more evidence is needed, it's important to pay attention to the data. My advice is if you don't want to take the risk, then don't get injectables. It's that simple. I am always wary of people who preach about something being harmful to one's health when it's not proven. It is your job as a patient to vet the information and make the best decision for yourself—not to listen to fearmongers—even if they are well intended.

"In retrospect, I wish I had done fillers in the middle of my treatment so I didn't get so hollow by the end," says Dr. Waldorf. "Some oncos let me do that for their patients—and I can tell you—it makes a huge difference."

Dr. Day agrees. "What doctors miss with these things is how much it supports your immune system when you feel better about yourself," she says. "When you look better, you feel better and when you feel better your immune system is stronger and you withstand stress better. Having that hope and feeling good have a great value and it's not just vanity. It doesn't make you less caring or serious about your treatment. One doesn't cancel out the other."

radiated skin: feeling the burn

What is radiation treatment? Radiation therapy uses high-energy X-rays to damage or kill cancer cells by preventing them from growing or dividing. Unlike chemotherapy, which uses drugs that have a systematic or whole-body effect, radiation therapy targets cancer cells in a localized area for a more focused treatment approach.

While the two treatments are very different, they share one important similarity: Both chemotherapy drugs and radiation X-rays can't distinguish between cancer cells and healthy cells and, ultimately, kill both.

"I always say the X-rays are not smart enough to know what is a cancer cell and what's a normal cell," says Dr. Michele Halyard, professor of radiation oncology at the Mayo Clinic and the interim dean of the Mayo Medical School. "So the radiation damages the cells' ability to repair themselves and to continue to divide and grow and replenish themselves. Basically, radiation causes damage in the tissue."

The course of radiation is dependent on a variety of things including the type of cancer, its location, and the number of treatments and dose level needed. Typically, breast cancers are treated with radiation for six weeks while skin cancer can be as short as a ten-day stint. The side effects can range from mild redness to the look and feel of a third-degree burn. It can also leave the tissue firmer and a different color than it was before treatment.

"Part of the other thing that is important to mention is, it's how the beams are delivered to the area that we need to treat that also determines the skin reaction," says Dr. Halyard. "With prostate cancer, for example, sometimes we have multiple angles of the X-ray beam coming in toward the prostate. So it's spreading the dose coming in at multiple different directions. So any direction doesn't necessarily get the full skin dose. With the breast, we have generally two or three beams coming in depending on how much of the volume you need to treat, so more of that dose may be coming to the skin."

For breast cancer patients who get six weeks of daily radiation treatments, side effects will start halfway through at about three weeks. For Caucasian patients, that will display itself in erythema or a pinkness of the skin—something that looks a lot like a sunburn—and is caused by basal dilation, when the capillaries are more open. Patients that have black or brown skin tones, who have more melanin, will start to see tanning or blackening of the skin. "For breast cancer we need to purposefully bring the full dose up to the skin surface, so by the end of treatment patients might experience moist desquamation, which is kind of a fancy name for a burn," says Dr. Halyard.

Treating the skin when it's compromised and stressed requires more than your average cream. Here's what Dr. Halyard and the Mayo Clinic advises patients try:

* **Get a Smart Start:** At the beginning of treatment, apply, daily, a hydrocortisone cream or a higher-percentage steroid cream like mometasone (1 percent hydrocortisone). "We've actually done what we call a cancer control trial at Mayo where it shows that in certain circumstances, patients may have less skin reaction with using some steroid up front [at the onset of treatment]," says Dr. Halyard.

* **Early On, Opt for Soothing Products:** Aloe vera gel and calendula lotion help soothe the skin while helping it retain moisture. Just steer clear of scent-based lotions that "dry the skin out," says Dr. Halyard.

* **Break Out the Big Guns for the Burn:** "Once you've got the denuding of the top layer of the skin cells, which looks like a burn, switch to products like Silvadene," says Dr. Halyard. The water-miscible cream contains the antimicrobial agent silver sulfadiazine in a micronized form that helps treat and prevent bacterial infections in second- and third-degree burns. "In our department at Mayo we'll sometimes use Aquaphor with Versalon gauze sponge pads, which are impregnated with a medication that helps in the healing of the skin." Other products that also do a good job:

  • **Desitin:** The diaper rash ointment contains maximum levels of zinc oxide, a mild astringent and antiseptic, that keeps the skin emollient and forms a protective barrier that encourages burn and wound healing.

  • **Biafine:** The topical, water-based emulsion increases the levels of macrophage cells, the immune cells, which aid in the three phases of healing: inflammation, proliferation, and maturation.

tip: stay cool and calm

Feeling the burn from radiation or have skin irritation from chemo? Here's an instant soother. "Take a wet cold compress and put a tablespoon of white vinegar on it," advises Dr. Richey. "The acidic element neutralizes the burning effect considerably." After, pat dry, then apply a little aloe vera or moisturizing cream.

what to avoid during radiation

* **Not All Ointments Are Created Equal:** While most of us are programmed to slather ointments like bacitracin and neomycin on our cuts or burns, this is one time you shouldn't. Dr. Halyard shares, "I've seen patients use Neosporin or Polysporin because they think it's going to help but—and I've not seen scientific evidence with this—anecdotally, to me, I've seen that they make skin reactions worse."

* **Certain Medications:** "Make sure you go over your medication list with your doctor to make sure you're not taking any drug that is photosensitizing; meaning that they make you more sensitive to the sun and cause redness in the skin," she advises. "Those drugs can also make you more sensitive to a skin reaction during radiation. Hydrochlorothiazide and thiazide-type diuretics are two examples."

* **Hold Off on Topical and Supplemental Antioxidants:** Radiation oxidizes the DNA in the skin cells creating what we call "free radicals." Antioxidants help keep the cells—both healthy and cancer cells—alive and abundant. "If you are taking or applying antioxidants, it defeats the purpose of radiation," says Dr. Halyard. "I have patients go off supplemental and topical antioxidants during their therapy." Better safe than sorry.

tip: get off the scent

"Use unscented laundry detergent and fabric softeners while in treatment," says Dr. Richey. "The scent and perfumes on them can drive skin crazy."

get the 411

Before you even begin your radiation treatment, try to gather as much information as you can from your doctor to prepare for what's to come. "Make sure you know going in what to expect," Dr. Halyard advises. Sit down with your radiation oncologist and get the 411 on what they anticipate your side effects will be, what you can do to help prevent and minimize them, and what their game plan will be in case you have any reactions. Additionally, during your therapy, you will have weekly on-treatment visits with your doctor and their nursing team. "Make sure they look at your skin and check it," she advises, so they are aware of any changes and can handle them promptly. Being aware, informed, and proactive, will benefit you—and your skin.

skin care *after* treatment
putting your best face forward

So, remember how I told you that you shouldn't use certain ingredients like antioxidants and retinols during treatment? Well, that was then and this is now. Once surgery, chemo, and radiation are in your rearview window and you've gotten the "all clear" from your docs—then you should start using potent products and treatments to get your skin to where it used to be. For those whose treatment or cancer drugs will put them into chemopause (medically induced menopause), a few power products will help prevent or minimize potential changes that will occur.

There isn't one particular regimen that will work for everyone. You're going to have to try a few things to see what works best for your needs. I suggest that as your treatment is winding down—before you begin taking any medication that will put you into meno-pause—that you make an appointment to see your dermatologist. He or she will be able to customize a skin care plan based on your specific issues and write prescriptions for products that are more powerful than anything you can buy over the counter.

That said, there are some things you should always have stocked in your medicine cabinet and some key ingredients to put in the mix. Let's start with ingredients to look for. The ones listed below are the most efficient and effective ingredients that will help transform aging or compromised skin.

top topical antioxidants

Earlier in this book, I described antioxidants as skin care heroes because they rescue our skin from many damaging elements includ-ing harmful UVA/UVB rays, free-radical damage, and the natural aging process. As we get older, our skin gets thinner and less resil-ient. Antioxidants, which are often formulated into our serums, eye creams, and moisturizers, help turn back time. Here are some of the most potent ones to get into the mix:

vitamin E

How it works: Vitamin E is a fat-soluble vitamin found naturally in the skin as well as many food sources. It helps the skin look younger by protecting cell membranes from oxidative damage, upping collagen levels, which plump fine lines and wrinkles (score!). What's interesting about vitamin E is that, unlike other vitamins, the skin derives more benefits from topical applications than through oral supplements. It comes in two forms: alpha-tocopherol (alcohol-based) and alpha-tocopherol acetate. The latter does not penetrate the skin as easily so make sure to read ingredient labels carefully to ensure you are getting the most bang for your buck.

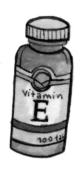

What to look for: Vitamin E, tocopherol, or tocotrienols.

resveratrol

How it works: Resveratrol is a potent polyphenolic antioxidant that is commonly found in grapes, blueberries, nuts, and red wine (I like this one for obvious reasons!). Studies have shown that when applied topically, resveratrol protects against UVB-mediated cutaneous damage and inhibits UVB-mediated oxidative stress. I call it the great protector because, when applied topically, it shields the skin from sun damage, reduces cell damage, and amps up collagen production. It also has amazing anti-inflammatory properties that can help with rosacea or acne-prone skin.

What to look for: Resveratrol or trihydroxystilbene.

vitamin B

How it works: This powerful antioxidant exhibits anti-inflammatory and depigmenting properties. It has also been shown to improve the texture and tone of the skin, as well as reduce fine lines, wrinkles, and hyperpigmentation.

What to look for: Vitamin B or niacinamide.

vitamin C

How it works: This is an essential nutrient that can only come from the fruits and veggies that contain it. Touted for its cold-fighting powers, it also works wonders at minimizing wrinkles, nixing dull skin, and reversing brown spots. Research also shows that it helps strengthen the skin's barrier response, enhancing the skin's repair process, reducing inflammation, and helping the skin withstand exposure to sunlight even if it's not protected by sunscreen! It's nothing short of a miracle worker. To get the best results, look for vitamin C products with a concentration of 5 to 20 percent packaged in a container that protects the formula from light and air. I love individual, single-use capsules. They keep the antioxidant stable while dosing out the right amount and are perfect for traveling.

What to look for: Vitamin C, L-ascorbic acid, or tetrahexyldecyl ascorbate.

retinol

How it works: Most people think of retinol as an acid because of its power to speed up cell turnover and exfoliate the skin. However, "retinol" is the general term for the entire vitamin A molecule. Most people know it because of Retin-A, the potent prescription cream that works for a host of skin-related issues, including acne and wrinkles. Regardless of the name or strength, it is a cell-communicating ingredient and antioxidant whose benefits are many. Retinol has been shown to increase the skin's collagen production and glycosaminoglycan content (a substance naturally found in young skin) resulting in firmer skin with improved texture and enhanced barrier function. It is also helpful for those with rosacea because it works against the inflammation caused by persistent redness and irritation.

What to look for: In over-the-counter products, it's found in the form of retinol, retinyl palmitate, and retinaldehyde. In prescription products, it's retinoic acid or tretinoin.

alpha hydroxy and beta hydroxy acids

How they work: What's the difference between alpha or beta hydroxy, you ask? The main difference is the lipid (oil) solubility. Alpha hydroxy acids are water-soluble, while beta hydroxy acid is oil-soluble. This means that beta hydroxy acid is able to penetrate into the pore that contains sebum and exfoliate the dead skin cells that are built up inside the pore. Beta hydroxy acid is better for oily skin that is prone to blemishes. Alpha hydroxy acids are better on sun-damaged or dry skin.

What to look for: Alpha hydroxy acids (sometimes listed as AHAs), glycolic acid, lactic acid, tartaric acid, malic acid, and citric acid. Beta hydroxy acid can also be listed as salicylic acid.

hyaluronic acid

How it works: This sugar-related molecule called a glycosaminoglycan is the body's lubricant molecule and is central to regulating cell growth and cell renewal. Hyaluronic acid has been called the "foundation of youth" because of its unique ability to bind with water—up to a thousand times its weight! Because it is a large, slippery molecule, it can't be absorbed into the skin but sits on the surface instead. This allows the water that it holds or attracts to remain on the surface as well, keeping the skin hydrated and smooth.

What to look for: Hyaluronic acid, hyaluronan, or hyaluronate.

lactobionic acid

How it works: This patented nonirritating "bionic" polyhydroxy acid derived from milk sugar helps prevent and reverse the appearance of photoaging, including lines and wrinkles, uneven pigment, enlarged pores, and roughness.

What to look for: Lactobionic acid or galactosylgluconic acid.

revving up your regimen

Knowing what ingredients can help with your skin is a good starting point. From there, you can look for those ingredients in specific products—like retinol in your night cream or vitamin C in your serum. There are so many variables that will come into play here—from skin type, skin issues, and skin goals—so I will keep it simple. Below is a short list of power products that are transformative for skin that's been compromised, damaged, or is feeling the effects of menopause-inducing meds. They include:

* Serum

* Eye cream

* Moisturizer

* Retinol-based night cream

* Sunblock

* Balm—lip and body

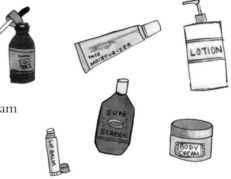

As a former beauty editor and director and now a TV beauty producer, I am lucky that I get to test virtually every brand on the market. Over the years, I have found that the cost of a product doesn't always indicate its quality. There are many expensive creams that celebrities rave about that I don't think live up to the hype. On the flip side, there are many drugstore brands that prevent me from looking like a shriveled hag. Ultimately, it comes down to what works for you. Personally, I prefer the skin care products that are science-based and evidence-backed. Besides the brands and products that I have recommended earlier in this chapter, the ones that follow have never let me down. These are the big guns that give my skin that extra oomph when it's showing signs of fatigue and age.

RoC: I live for this drugstore brand! The Retinol Correxion Sensitive Night Cream is formulated with a mild retinol and hyaluronic acid so it's perfect for beginners or those with sensitive skin. It delivers serious results without leaving the skin flaky or peeling. Plus, it won't break the bank—costing roughly £25. If you want to take it up a notch, the Deep Wrinkle Night Cream is the way to go. Every time I use it, I wake up with skin that is glowing and youthful.

Neocutis: When my Tamoxifen started to show itself in the form of wrinkles around my eyes, I turned to Neocutis Lumière Bio-Restorative Eye Balm for its *Benjamin Button*–like abilities. No matter how many hours I have worked or how few hours I have slept, a few dabs of this eye cream makes me look bright-eyed and bushy-tailed. It contains caffeine, hyaluronic acid, and bisabolol that hydrates the delicate skin under the eyes, diminishes dark circles and depuffs almost instantly. Neocutis works off precise Swiss technology and cellular research, which inevitably leads them to scientifically advanced breakthroughs. Their latest line Micro Essentials, powered by Micro Protein Complex, uses synthetic peptides to turn back the clock without growth factors. "I use their micro eye product because it has newer, more potent technology," says Dr. Waldorf. "I also like the Micro Essentials Micro-Day cream. It has the micropeptide technology, antioxidants and sun protection, so it's a great all-in-one."

Revision Skincare: Most people have not heard of Revision, but it's a small brand that has made a big impression on me. The first time I experienced the results of their D-E-J eye cream was when a colleague of mine asked if I had an eye cream to help with her dark under-eye bags. I gave her this cream from the beauty closet and promptly forgot about it. A few days later, she came back to my office with skin that was so smooth and even-toned it looked airbrushed. The transformation to the delicate skin under her eyes was almost shocking. Key ingredients include vitamin C, copper, and palmitoyl tripeptide-38.

SkinCeuticals: Their tagline "Advanced Skincare Backed by Science" pretty much says it all. Known for their potent serums and age-defying creams, this brand is for those who take their skin care seriously. Ironically, this line was born from decades of skin cancer research, which led to pivotal breakthroughs in concentrated antioxidants. Sandra Lee and I are huge fans of the brand and made them a cornerstone of our post-cancer skin care regimens. "The C E Ferulic topical antioxidant is the bomb," Sandra says. "After I wake up I put this stuff all over my face and neck. It makes me look thirty again. So, I live on it."

NeoStrata: This dermatologist-developed brand is known for their advancements in therapeutic and cosmetic products whose formulas are based in polyhydroxy acid technology. They target and treat issues including acne, hyperkeratosis, and extremely dry skin. One of their hero products, the Bionic Face Serum, lives up to its name. The key ingredients, polyhydroxy acid and lactobionic acid, perform just like traditional alpha hydroxy acids; however, because they are larger molecules, they are gentler and cause less peeling, flaking, and dryness. The results include brighter skin, smaller pores, and a baby-soft feel.

MD Complete: This is one brand that I really love and support. The line of products contains high concentrations of hardworking ingredients, specifically lab-crafted micro peptides, which are potent but not irritating. I also love that the brand supports Dr. Donald Richey's Brighter Days program, which helps cancer patients deal with the dermatological side effects of their treatment. Word on the street is that they are developing a product line that is specifically for cancer patients. I can't wait to see what this dynamic duo creates.

the great debate: growth factors

There is one final ingredient that I want to chat about before closing out this chapter: human growth factors (HGFs). These are proteins produced by the body that act as chemical messengers. They bind to the surface of a cell and then instruct that cell to activate the production of new cells, and to grow or divide into cells with different functions. Originally, HGFs were utilized in wound healing to stimulate collagen production and repairing damaged skin—especially with second- and third-degree burns. After seeing the impressive results the HGFs yielded, skin care brands started utilizing them as well. Today, they have become a popular ingredient in antiaging skin care.

While this all sounds amazing, there are some very real concerns that HGFs used in certain concentrations and durations can cause cells to overproliferate. While this is the point in wound healing, the risk is that they can accelerate the growth of skin cancer by stimulating the overproduction of sleeper skin cancer cells. There are some derms that believe that a cocktail with HGFs mixed in are unlikely to have a stimulatory effect on cancer cells. But other experts, including New York City–based dermatologist Dr. Jeannette Graf, believe the uncertainty is too risky—especially for those who have had cancer. "Human growth factors can start out as the good guys, the wound healers. By the time they communicate with every single receptor, they can wake up sleeper cells that end up as tumor promoters," says Dr. Graf, the author of *Stop Aging, Start Living*. "That's why I'm very, very careful." She continues the thought: "When using a powerful product with HGF that can stimulate wound healing, you have to ask, 'What else is it doing?' I can't answer that because I have not seen much science on it."

I am a firm believer in doing what you think is best for you, while using precaution. But crow's-feet versus skin cancer seems like a no-brainer. Before you use any skin care products, make sure you know what ingredients the formula contains so you can make an educated decision about what you are putting on your skin and into your body.

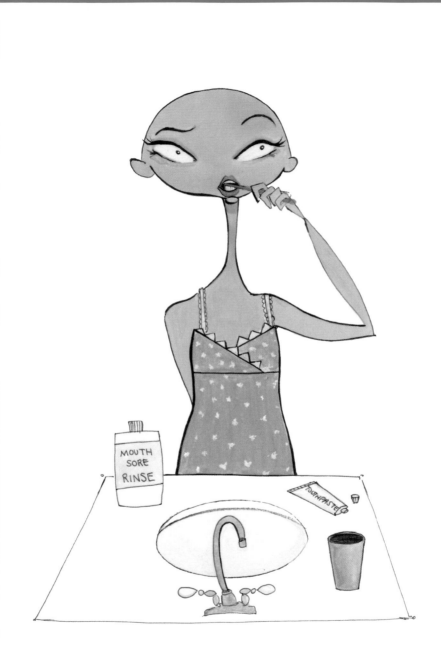

CHAPTER 4

GETTING MOUTHY

let's chat about oral care

One of things most cancer patients don't expect they will have to deal with during treatment is oral care. I mean, who the hell is thinking about flossing and rinsing when you just had your breast cut into and a chunk of your hair is lying on the bathroom floor? I barely got to the dentist on a regular basis when I was healthy, so when I got sick, it was the furthest thing from my mind. Regardless, oral mucositis (mouth sores), xerostomia (dry mouth), and oral thrush affect up to 40 percent of patients having chemotherapy and almost every patient that undergoes radiation. These oral care issues can have serious implications on a patient's health and need to be given proper attention.

In the same way that chemotherapy and radiation target and kill rapidly dividing cells that lead to hair loss and dry skin, they also cause canker sores and cotton-mouth. I know, it bites!

"Chemotherapy causes cell death and in the oral cavity it makes the mucosal lining thin. It may slough off, become red, inflamed, and ulcerated causing mouth sores," says Dr. Brian Kantor, cosmetic dentist and partner in Lowenberg Lituchy & Kantor in Manhattan. "With radiation, the salivary glands are affected and produce less saliva. So the mouth is less lubricated and becomes very dry."

Both issues can be debilitating in their own way. The biggest issue with mouth sores—which can get as large as one and a half inches in some cases—is that they can make eating so painful that patients consume less and their nutrition becomes compromised. Malnourishment weakens the immune system, which

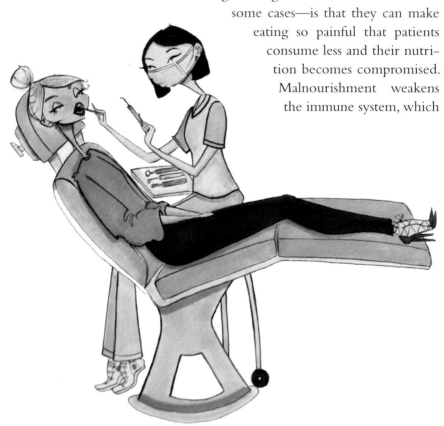

slows down the body's ability to fight infection and heal. A lack of protein and calories also affect your energy level, which we all know is critical for maintaining the stamina required for this type of battle.

Dry mouth doesn't seem as problematic but is it. Here's why: "Saliva acts as a lubricant but it does so much more than that," says Dr. Kantor. "Saliva contains enzymes that break down bacteria that cause cavities. It helps wash away food debris so it's not sticking to your teeth creating bacteria and causing decay." In many ways, saliva is like an antibiotic for the body because it acts as an infection fighter— something especially critical for cancer patients.

the *first* piece of advice is this...

Before you start chemo or radiation it is imperative that you go see your dentist. Now, I know what you are thinking: "I am basically living in doctors' offices and you want me to make *another* appointment to see my *dentist*?!" Yes. That is exactly what I'm saying. Ideally, you should see your dentist a month before you start treatment but since time isn't always on our side with these things, just try to get there as soon as possible. The reason it's so important is this: "Cancer patients are prone to infections when going through chemo and if you already have an abscess or something, it's going to get much worse," says Dr. Kantor. "It's better to take care of it beforehand." When you schedule your checkup, also schedule a cleaning. Having clean, healthy teeth won't cause infections that interrupt, delay, or pause your treatments later on.

Okay—so let's chat about how to prevent or minimize these nasty side effects.

dry mouth

There are a few things you can do ensure dry mouth doesn't become a larger, problematic issue:

* **Drink up:** Make sure you are getting the recommended eight eight-ounce glasses of water a day. If you are not a fan of aqua, like me, then you're going to have to get creative with flavoring it. I squeeze a slice of Meyer lemon (a cross between a lemon and a Mandarin orange) into every glass, otherwise, I just can't get it down. For me, this hybrid fruit gives the water a citrusy-sweet taste that helps me enjoy it. If you are experiencing upset stomach or acid reflux during treatment, avoid acidic fruits like lemon, grapefruit, orange, and lime. Instead, make some fruit-and veggie-infused "spa water"—like the kind you drink before a massage. There are a million different recipes for them—most of which are delicious and taste more like a cocktail. My top three faves: cucumber 'n' mint, watermelon 'n' rosemary and pineapple 'n' strawberry.

* **Suck it:** "Chewing ice is bad for your teeth," says Dr. Kantor. "But sucking on a piece of ice actually helps lubricate the mouth." It also helps prevent mouth sores. "Right before my infusions would start, the nurses would give me a plastic cup of ice chips," says Joan Lunden, legendary newswoman and survivor of stage II triple negative breast cancer. "I would put them in my mouth and roll them around for five minutes. It chills all the blood vessels and keeps the chemo from going into those blood vessels. It definitely prevents those horrible mouth sores." To make the experience more enjoyable, suck on your favorite Popsicle or freeze some flavored water. Then you will please your taste buds while keeping your mouth moist and healthy.

* **Reach for a rinse:** There are a few mouth rinses that can alleviate the feeling that you have a piece of sandpaper in your mouth, rather than a tongue. They include:

- **Biotene:** This over-the-counter rinse was created with cancer patients in mind and is the number one recommended dry mouth treatment by the Oral Cancer Foundation. And here's why: The alcohol-free rinse is formulated with ingredients that lubricate the mouth for up to four hours. It also helps balance the pH of the mouth and keeps it clean. The rinse can be used up to five times a day.

- **PerioSciences:** In the past, most oral care brands would use alcohol in their products to kill bacteria and hydrogen peroxide to help brighten teeth. However, research shows that there are real issues with both ingredients. While alcohol kills off bacteria, it also dries out the oral tissue, which inadvertently becomes a breeding ground for bacteria. Hydrogen peroxide, on the other hand, triggers oxidative stress, which causes inflammation in the mouth. Both ingredients are too harsh for patients in treatment. PerioSciences is an oral care company that formulates their products—including their AO ProRinse and Dry Mouth AO Pro Gel—with natural antioxidants and polyphenol ingredients that work in tandem with the saliva's antimicrobial agents. The formula is gentle on the tissue but pretty potent when it comes to keeping the mouth hygienic and healthy. It's important to note that PerioSciences was not intended for cancer patients. Dentists who saw the positive results the rinse and gel yielded began recommending it for off-label purposes—for patients experiencing cotton-mouth during chemotherapy or radiation treatments. I used it for a brief time during my treatment and it made a huge difference. Because it's intended to maintain a healthy mouth, the sooner you can start using before treatment, the better.

mouth *sores*

If you've ever had a canker sore, you know what a nightmare mouth sores can be. The first line of defense is an easy, old-school fix: a warm saltwater rinse. Saline helps disinfect aphthous ulcers and minimize inflammation. Here's how to make one from stuff in your kitchen:

* Mix a teaspoon or two of salt with a glass of warm water. (If you don't have salt handy or if you can't handle the taste, use a pinch of baking soda instead.)

* Hold the mixture in your mouth and swish from side to side.

* After three minutes, spit it out in the sink. Try not to swallow it, as the salt can make you dehydrated.

* Repeat after meals and before bed.

If this saline mixture doesn't do the trick, "There's something called Magic Mouthwash and this is what I give to all my patients that have sores," says Dr. Kantor. "This soothes the mouth and enables patients to eat and talk. It doesn't take the sores away but it takes the pain away." So, what is Magic Mouthwash? It is a mouthwash that your doctor or dentist has to prescribe for a pharmacist to make. There are two variations. The basic recipe is below:

magic mouthwash recipe

300 cc of Benadryl

60 cc of Mylanta

4 g of Carafate

For cases where the sores are severe and painful, the pharmacist will add viscous lidocaine, a numbing medication, to the recipe. For those who get the lidocaine formula, it's important to shake the mouthwash well before taking. Some patients who forgot reported their head or mouth being numb for longer than expected.

Magic Mouthwash used to be a pretty common concoction that pharmacists would make. Today, it has taken a backseat to more convenient over-the-counter topical treatments and painkillers. "I would say 20 to 30 percent of the time, the pharmacy will call and tell me they don't know what it is or that they don't know the ingredients. Once I give it to them, its no problem," say Dr. Kantor. "It's still one of the most effective treatments, so I still prescribe it to my patients."

brush up your technique

We all know brushing your teeth is key to keeping your mouth healthy. If you're like me, you squeeze a teetering heap of toothpaste onto your brush, then go to town scrubbing off every bit of plaque and grime that might have accumulated on your chompers during the day or overnight. This isn't exactly the best way to brush—especially if you are experiencing mouth sensitivities. So, let's review the proper technique:

1 **Soften up:** It imperative to use an extra-soft tooth-brush. "Platelets decrease during chemo so the blood doesn't clot as fast," says Dr. Kantor. Gentle bristles equal less bleeding.

2 **Warm up:** "The trick is to soak the bristles in very hot water for a minute before brushing," he advises. "The extra soft bristles become even softer in the hot water so they are not so abrasive on the gums."

3 **Angle down:** Most of us brush our teeth from side to side or back and forth. That movement is too abrasive for teeth. It wears down the enamel and rubs along the sensitive gums. The gentlest technique is to hold your toothbrush at a forty-five-degree angle and brush downward.

get *flossy*

With all this info about decreased platelets, sensitive gums, and mouth sores—you're probably thinking that flossing isn't such a smart idea. It's actually just the opposite. Because cancer patients are prone to infection, it's critical to make sure you are removing any residue and bacteria that may linger between your teeth.

"You have to floss," says Dr. Kantor. "Even though it hurts—you have to floss." Here's why: Brushing and rinsing alone won't clean all the areas in your mouth. Between the teeth is the hardest area to clean and the only way you can do that is to floss. If you're not flossing, you're not cleaning those areas, and if you're not cleaning those areas, you're leaving yourself open to possible infections—ones that are harder to fight when your immune system is compromised. Why take that risk?

toothpaste

When I was going through treatment, I thought toothpaste for sensitive teeth was the best way to protect my tender mouth. It is if you have sensitive teeth. It won't help if you have sensitive gums. I'm going to blame that dumb choice on my chemo brain. While most toothpaste is gentle enough, Dr. Kantor suggests avoiding whitening toothpastes that are formulated with silicone and abrasives.

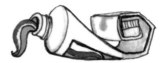

eat, drink, and be *merry!*

It's hard to talk about the mouth and not talk about what goes in it—food! For many of us in treatment, food takes on a love-hate relationship. Nausea, change in smell, and stress affect how much we can tolerate. But we still need to eat. It can make the battle more challenging, for sure.

While researching the chapter on scent for this book, I came across an intriguing study, "Learned Food Aversions in Children Receiving Chemotherapy." Published in 1978 in the *Journal of Science*, the study was conducted by Dr. Ilene Bernstein, a neuroscientist and psychology professor at the University of Washington. I believe her findings are so significant, they should be universally adopted into all aspects of cancer care.

Let me fill you in. You know what a food aversion is, right? It's when we eat too much of one thing and get sick from it or we taste something that repulses us and we develop a dislike for it. That is "learned taste aversion." Dr. Bernstein's study began as a way to see if pediatric cancer patients were developing aversions to their foods in relation to their treatment. She set out to conduct a sensitive test that could be evaluated.

"Everyone knows that children are incredibly food neophobic. They don't like to try new things," says Dr. Bernstein. "And children coming in for chemotherapy are even less likely to want to taste something novel before their chemo. So the question was, 'What do you give a child that they will be unlikely to turn down?' And the answer came to us: ice cream."

To ensure the flavor was novel, Dr. Bernstein enlisted an ice cream manufacturer in town to create an unusual flavor. She didn't want it to be unpleasant, but one that children normally wouldn't order. That flavor was Maple Puff—a unique mixture of maple and black walnuts. "We had them come back several weeks later and we offered them the ice cream. If they had the ice cream before they had chemotherapy, they didn't want it again. If they had the ice cream before a regular checkup, the were perfectly happy to eat it again."

The study proved that the one group who had an association between the ice cream flavor and their chemotherapy symptoms actually avoided eating the ice cream again.

So, how can cancer patients put this intel to work for them during treatment? I asked Dr. Bernstein.

"One approach is to sequester some foods that you never consume before chemo," she advises. For example, if pizza is your all-time favorite food, it's probably best to hold off eating it the day of your treatments. "You want to safeguard the dishes you really love from becoming associated with chemo later on."

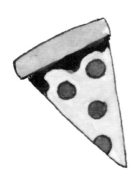

Interestingly enough, in follow-up studies, Dr. Bernstein found that foods with strong odors and protein seemed more likely to become targets of aversions over other nutrients. Also on the "no fly list"— spicy and acidic foods, alcohol, sugar, and caffeine. Bland foods including mashed potatoes, chicken soup, plain pasta, and gravies are the way to go.

speaking of *eating...*

* In the same way that Popsicles are great for children who have sore throats or have just had their teeth pulled, Popsicles will help soothe your mouth by helping to take down some of the inflammation and to numb the mouth a bit. I suggest making your own with organic natural, nonacidic juices like apple juice, guava, mango, peach. Avoid things that are acidic, like oranges, which will have the opposite effect.

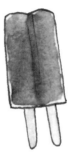

* Smoothies are also a nice way to get your supplements and nutrients in a way that won't be irritating to your mouth or stomach.

* Sorbets and frozen yogurt made with some dairy is a yummy way to load up on your vitamin D and calcium.

* Freezing small fruits like grapes is a great way to soothe the mouth and get nutrients at the same time. You can suck on them to reduce inflammation and irritations while also loading up on vitamins B_6, K, thiamin, and riboflavin.

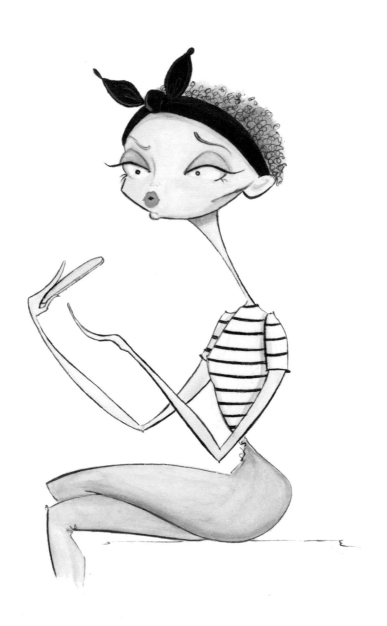

CHAPTER 5

STAY POLISHED

nail treatments you need to know about

At this point in the book you know that chemotherapy targets and kills rapidly dividing cells without discriminating against those that are healthy or cancerous. It's what causes hair loss, dry skin, mouth sores   and yes—even dramatic nail changes.

"It's the one side effect that no one expects, but the nails are the windows to your health," says my friend and celebrity manicurist, Elle Gerstein. Her clients include an endless roster of A-listers including Blake Lively, Angelina Jolie, and Jennifer Lopez (whom she has worked on for over eighteen years!). During my treatment, I turned to Elle for advice on how to care for my nails.

As she said, "It's the first telltale sign that something is going wrong with your body."

She's right about this. For me, the sign of my illness revealed itself in my nails long before I felt my lump. Almost two years before my diagnosis, my thumbnails began growing with extremely deep horizontal ridges and indentations in them. They were so deep, I would aggressively buff down the top surface, then drip ridge-filling basecoat into the crevices before polishing. While I knew that buffing the top of the nail was one of the most damaging things I could do, I was desperate to have pretty fingertips. Since I hadn't gotten my hand slammed in a car door, experienced a shock or traumatic event six month earlier (one of the supposed causes of ridges in the nail), I was really at a loss about what was causing this problem. When I was diagnosed with cancer, one of the oncologic surgeons that I interviewed asked me how long I had had the ridges in my nails. She explained that nail health is often a mirror of one's overall health. Fast-forward to today, my nails are fragile and peeling (thanks, menopause!), but the nail plate is smooth and relatively normal.

Nails are resilient structures and can endure a tremendous amount of trauma. That's why many people who go through chemotherapy won't lose their nails or won't show any signs of stress. But a lot of that depends on the type of chemotherapy drugs you receive. According to the American Cancer Society:

The most common chemo drugs used for early breast cancer include the anthracyclines (such as doxorubicin/Adriamycin and epirubicin/Ellence) and the taxanes (such as paclitaxel/Taxol and docetaxel/Taxotere). These may be used in combination with certain other drugs, like fluorouracil (Adrucil), cyclophosphamide (Cytoxan), and carboplatin. For cancers that are HER2 positive, the targeted drug trastuzumab (Herceptin) is often given with one of the taxanes. Pertuzumab (Perjeta) can also be combined with trastuzumab and docetaxel for HER2 positive cancers.

Docetaxel and paclitaxel are a part of the taxane group and probably the most devastating for the nails. A study conducted in 2005 revealed that the overall incidence of taxane-induced nail changes is as high as 44 percent. Another study, "Nail Toxicities Induced by Systemic Anticancer Treatments" published in *The Lancet* in April 2015, yielded similar results but went further, reporting that women who experienced nail changes stated that "this adverse side effect was the most unpleasant side effect."

Chemotherapy-induced nail changes are not pretty—that's for sure. They include:

* Paronychia (a tender bacterial or fungal infection in the skin surrounding the nail)

* Beau's lines (transverse grooves on the nail plate)

* Decreased linear nail growth and thickness

* Melanonychia (hyperpigmention or discoloration)

* Subungual hematomas (bleeding under the nail)

* Pseudomonas superinfections (pus-filled infections)

* Onycholysis (separation of the nail plate from the nail bed)

* Periungual lesions (lesions around the nails)

* Loss of moisture

* Loss of elasticity

* Discoloration

* Nail loss

What sets these side effects apart from those of the skin and hair is that they aren't immediate. Since nails grow at a slow rate, under one millimeter per day, it takes almost two months for the nails that were formed during the early days of chemo to grow out long enough to be seen. (It's even slower for toes—but oddly—chemo typically doesn't affect the nails on your feet. Crazy, right?) While it may be slightly comforting that these changes are temporary, that's still not much of a consolation for those of us who considered ourselves beauty junkies. Not wear the latest nail color? Not an option!

The bad news is that the nail changes caused by chemo can't be fixed by any special treatments. Why? Because the damage to the matrix (the part of the nail that is responsible for producing cells that become the nail plate) formed months before it became visible, so there is nothing you can do to reverse the damage now. There are, however, things you can do to improve how your fingertips look.

keep your tips dry

Water can be an irritant to the nail bed, nail plate, and to the skin. Nails that get wet repeatedly tend to be weaker and prone to peeling and breakage. Bacteria and infections also thrive in wet and damp environments. Rubber gloves will be your savior for wet work like cleaning

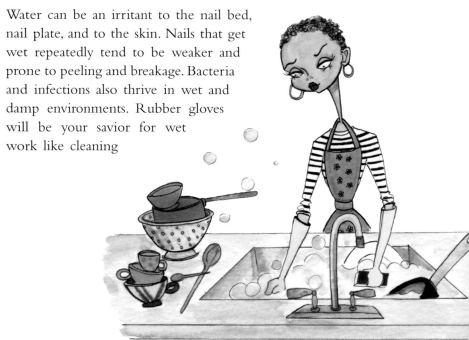

the dishes. If your nails are in really bad shape—e.g., nail loss, nail lifting—wear cotton gloves under the rubber gloves to help absorb any moisture and add a cushiony layer of protection.

break out the biotin

The only supplement with scientific evidence for achieving strong, healthy nails is biotin, a water-soluble B vitamin. Nail dermatologists typically recommend 2.5 milligrams a day.

get growing

Studies show that some topical treatments can be beneficial, especially for those suffering from fragile nails. "There are also two FDA approved prescription topical medications, Genadur [a hydro-soluble lacquer] and Nuvail [a polyurethane protective solution], that are formulated to help brittle, peeling, ridging, and split nails—nails that are fragile and prone to easy breakage," says Dr. Dana Stern, assistant clinical professor of dermatology at Icahn 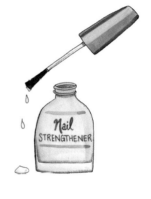 School of Medicine at Mount Sinai and the CEO-founder of Dr. Dana: Natural Nail Care System, the first dermatologist-created nail line. "Genadur contains an ingredient called hydroxypropyl chitosan (HPCH) that works by filling in the microscopic gaps within the nail surface to provide physical support and a barrier against external agents. Picture Teflon coating; it's a protective coating that prevents water from getting into the nail but still allows the nail to function. Polish can be applied over it. Nuvail is a similar concept. It creates a flexible structure within the nail plate, maintaining moisture balance and forms a sealant that protects the nail." (Make sure to talk to your oncologist before using any vitamins or topical medications.)

Two months after Dr. Stern put me on Genadur I saw an improvement in my nails. It was a subtle improvement, but an improvement nonetheless. Genadur is expensive, so ask your doctor to give you a tester bottle first to make sure it works before shelling out your hard-earned dough. Once I got a prescription for a full bottle, I was pleasantly surprised that it was covered by my insurance.

soak it up

Okay—so here's a gross fact. More than twenty different species of bacteria can be cultured from nail lesions. If you are experiencing this type of side effect, your dermatologist can prescribe an antiseptic soak that can help reduce bacteria and inflammation. "I usually use a boro solution, which is an over-the-counter aqueous water-based solution that contains aluminum acetate," says Dr. Stern. "It has astringent and antibacterial properties that are effective with these bacteria issues. But it's important to seek the care of your physician to deal with these types of side effects." Anything that involves infection should involve your doctor.

(not) tool time

One of the main reasons our nails peel and break is because we tend to use them as tools—like as a screwdriver or scraper. Be mindful of how you use your nails so that you can limit how much impact and trauma *you* inflict on them.

be gentle

Nail cosmetics—polishes, gels, decals—have a huge impact on the health of our nails. Remover is by far the harshest of them all. "Polish needs to be taken off with a strong solvent and normally in the salons they use acetone," says Dr. Stern. "It is extremely drying and dehydrating to the nail and exacerbates brittleness." To keep nails in tiptop shape, opt for acetone-free removers. Yeah, it may take longer to get your polish off, but your nails will thank you for it. The best acetone-free remover is Zoya Remove Plus. It takes off the most stubborn polish in one swipe. I've tried a lot of removers during my career as a beauty director and this is the only one I will use.

stock up on hand cream

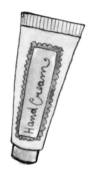

The main culprit behind dry hands and brittle nails is a lack of moisture. Keep a rich cream on hand at all times. Apply it liberally and often. My faves are: Neutrogena Norwegian Formula Hand Cream, Kiehl's Ultimate Strength Hand Salve, and L'Occitane Shea Intensive Hand Balm.

DIY manicures

Not to sound dramatic, but even the smallest infection can escalate into a much bigger problem—and quickly—when your immune system is compromised. While getting a mani-pedi is *normally* a great way to pamper yourself, it's a bit too risky while you are in treatment. Even in the cleanest salons, germs and bacteria linger everywhere. Foot soaks are exposed to an endless turnover of other people's nail clippings, shaved callus flakes, and toe crud. But that isn't the worst of it. In 2000, a physician in Northern California treated four patients with furunculosis caused by *Mycobacterium bolletii* and *M. massiliense*. All four patients had received pedicures at the same nail salon—and each ended up with pus-filled sores on their lower legs. In 2011, dermatologists at the University of North Carolina-Chapel Hill reported three similar cases—and you guessed it—all three patients had had pedicures at the same salon. The moral of the story is this: You're playing the odds when you soak your feet in public pedicure basins.

While some people will try to sell you on the idea that an at-home pedi can be as relaxing—I'm not one of them. It's less physically taxing when someone else clips and files your toenails. That said, I feared getting a case of foot fungus or an infection and just decided to take matters into my own hands (pun intended). I would try to make doing my nails as enjoyable as possible by making a "spa night" out of it. I would put on some chill music, make myself some cucumber- and mint-infused water (just like at the spa!) and would pick out a fun nail color to wear. If I were feeling really ambitious, I'd even put a face mask on, too. (I am obsessed with the Korean sheet masks!) Once I finished painting my nails, I'd plop myself in front of the TV and catch up on my favorite shows while they dried. This made it more indulgent than any nail salon—and it cost a heck of a lot less!

Over the years, I have interviewed Elle about her famous clients, the hottest trends, and how to master a salon-worthy mani at home. Now, she shares her pro tips for us Cancer Cuties, so we can get our weak, compromised nails in the best shape possible. Here's what she has to say:

snip 'n' clip

If you need to cut your nails before you file, make sure you are doing so with a nail clipper, NOT a toenail clipper. Using a larger clipper for a one-snip shortcut will cause the nail to snap. The proper way to cut the nail is in two separate clips so that it doesn't bend in the opposite (convex) direction and break. Clip from outer edge to the center, then again from the center to the opposite edge. If your nail is lifting off the skin (the nail bed), clip it down to where it is still attached. This will prevent it from snagging or tearing. If your nails are lifting in a way that is bothering you or if you have an open cut," says Elle, "wrap the finger in light, breathable gauze."

handle hangnails properly

If you have a hangnail, trim it so that it doesn't tear further. But make sure to wash and disinfect your hands immediately as the smallest tear in the skin can lead to an infection. Don't cut the cuticles either. The cuticle sits above the matrix, where the nail plate forms and acts as a bumper to protect the nail when it is first forming. If the cuticle has been cut, the newly formed nail will grow in weak and with ridges. Instead, use a cuticle stick with a rubber cushion tip to gently push back the skin and clean up the nail.

the file is key

Steer clear of abrasive files. If it feels rough, it's going to rough up your nails. Edges that are jagged and ragged will peel and break. Never use metal. Look for a file with a 240 to 600 grit. Elle and Dr. Stern are big fans of glass (also known as "crystal") files. They seal the keratin layers together at the edge of the nail, which prevents it from splitting and fraying. Filing the nail in a sawing motion may be the fastest way to get the job done but it also roughs up the free edge. "Filing in one direction is the most gentle way to do it," says Elle, adding, "Never, ever file the top or sides of the nail."

shape helps strength

"A lot of people like very square nails but square nails snag," says Elle. Most of us know there is nothing more painful than when the nail catches on something and tears. "When you are filing, make sure to round off the edges slightly."

cuticle oil heals

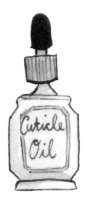

Hands down, the number-one thing for healthy nails is moisture. Nourished nails that have enough elasticity and flexibility won't snap and break. Applying cuticle oil will keep nails pliable and prevent delaminating, when the top layers separate from the lower layers of the nail. Oils formulated with vitamin E are the most hydrating, but those found in your kitchen—including coconut oil, sweet almond oil, jojoba oil, and olive oil—are just as hardy. Rubbing it on the cuticle to get the blood flowing will help stimulate cell regeneration and growth.

don't skip the base coat

It might be an annoying step, especially when you're tight on time, but using a base coat is super important. Those infused with peptides, keratin, and other hydrating ingredients strengthen and fortify the nail while protecting it from polish, impact, and environmental stressors.

pick a safe polish

Nail lacquers are made primarily of chemicals. One whiff and you know this is true. With a push from the public, more and more beauty companies are formulating their polishes as "3-Free," meaning they do not contain the "toxic trio" of chemicals: dibutyl phthalate (DBP), formaldehyde, and toluene. Other brands have gone even further, excluding formaldehyde resin

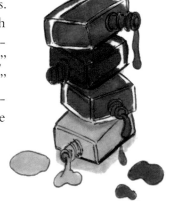

(tosylamide/TSFR) and camphor. When shopping or selecting polish, make sure you choose the healthiest and safest options, which are brands that are 3-, 4-, or 5-Free. My top picks include: Zoya, RGB, Essie, Butter London, Chanel, and Deborah Lippman. One of my favorite brands, Smith & Cult, formulates polishes that are 8-Free without sacrificing color, long-wear, or a high-shine finish!

finishing touches

Even if you don't feel like painting your nails, finishing off your mani with a topcoat will make a world of difference. Not only will it give your nails a glossy shine, it also helps bind the layers of the nail together and protect it from impact and outside elements.

tip: try this hot mani trick

If nails need some extra love, try weekly hot oil manicures. "Put a little cuticle oil on a cotton ball and put it on the tip of your finger, then cover with tin foil," says Doug Schoon, leading research scientist and product developer in the nail industry and president of Schoon Scientific. "Warm the foil with your hair dryer. The oil will penetrate much more quickly and deeply than it will at room temperature and helps reverse brittleness. It keeps the layers of the nails lubricated so they slide back and forth and won't snap."

cryotherapy

In the same way that cold caps help prevent hair loss, cryotherapy—an intervention using frozen gel gloves—preserves nails from cutaneous reactions or loss. It is primarily used on patients who are receiving docetaxel-infused chemotherapy. The way it works is "the cold temperature (of the gloves) causes vasoconstriction, which is when the blood vessels simply constrict and become smaller," says Dr. Stern. "This reduces the amount of the chemotherapy drug that reaches the nail or hair follicle, preventing toxicity."

Cryotherapy can reduce various chemo side effects, including nail disfigurement, blistering, desquamation, or shedding of the skin, pain, infections, and nail loss. A control study published in the American Society of Clinical Oncology in 2005 applied the frozen gel gloves fifteen minutes prior to the administration of docetaxel, during the hour-long infusion and fifteen minutes at the end of the infusion. The results of the study were impressive. Nail toxicities dropped from 51 percent to 11 percent and a nail loss flatlined at 0 percent in the gloved hand versus 22 percent in the unprotected hand.

While cryotherapy provides many patients with a solution to a very real and bothersome side effect, there are some downsides. Many patients can't tolerate the freezing feeling of the gloves. There are also some oncologists and hospitals that won't use it—the thought being that if the chemo isn't reaching a particular area of the body, then it can't kill cancer cells lurking there.

I am on the fence about this one. On one hand I feel like you should do everything you can to wipe cancer from your body and allow the chemo to its job—even if that means losing your nails. On the other hand, nobody knows more than me the importance of being able to retain a sense of self and normalcy during treatment. It's why I wrote this book. Ultimately, says Dr. Stern, "It's an individual decision that should be discussed with your oncologist." And I couldn't agree more.

A positive end note: While the side effects of chemotherapy may be hard to deal with, they are temporary. Six months or a year from now, all this nail drama will be but a memory. Until then, just do your best to show your nails love and keep them healthy.

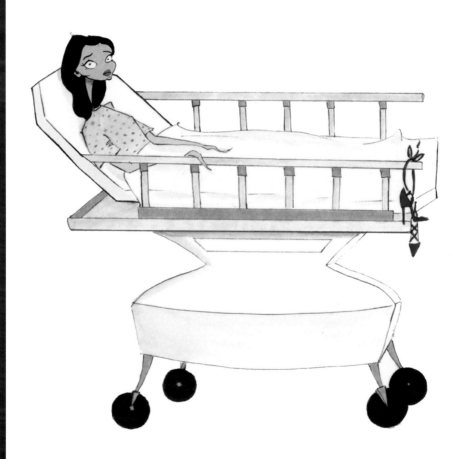

CHAPTER 6

TIT TALK

surgery and reconstruction

Today, there are more surgical options for cancer than ever before. This is especially true of breast cancer where removal of the tumor(s) and reconstruction vary on what I call the "Three Ps": the pathology, the patient, and the professional. Early on, breast cancer patients will face choices about their surgery and treatment. Depending on their type of cancer, they might also have to consider the type of reconstruction to opt for. If there is a silver lining to having breast cancer, it's that there are many reconstruction options and the results can be jaw-droppingly beautiful. Trust me when I say that it softens the blow. No matter what type of cancer you have, the decisions you make regarding the type of surgery and treatment will be a huge factor in your recovery. But they aren't the most important things you will have to decide on during this battle. This chapter explains my experience and that of those I have interviewed, however the process may differ depending on where you live and whether you have a private health care provider or are with the NHS. If you require more specific advice about surgery and reconstruction in your area please contact your GP or the Breast Cancer Care charity.

the *key* to it all: finding the best surgeon

Getting a cancer diagnosis makes you feel like you have been swept up in a tornado. And in a way, you have been. It knocks you off your feet and before you know it, you're whipping around from one doctor's office to another. For me, the most surprising part of this process was that the first doctor I was instructed to see was the surgical oncologist. "Why am I seeing a surgeon before seeing an oncologist?" I thought. It's a common question because it is the reverse of what happens with most illnesses. Typically, a patient goes to their primary medical doctor first, then to a specialist or surgeon. It's just the opposite when it comes to breast cancer. Surgery comes first because the size, location, and pathology of the tumor(s) often determine the subsequent treatment protocol that is necessary.

After finding out you have cancer, you are going to feel like you need to rush and get it removed STAT. This is very normal. In fact, I would be a little worried if you didn't feel that way. But before you work yourself into a panic, consider this: The probability is that you've most likely had this cancer for months, if not years, without even knowing it. Just to give you some perspective, my surgical oncologist told me that my one-inch tumor was probably growing for a few years before I felt it. So…taking a week or two isn't going to put you any further into the danger zone. In fact, the only thing that will put you there is getting any ol' doc to do the job.

Who you have as your surgeon is important because he/she paves the road for the rest of your cancer journey. Their experience and expertise will ensure that the cancer is removed from your body and that it is done in a way that takes your physical and emotional well-being into consideration. They may also make recommendations for the rest of your medical team, including your medical oncologist, radiology oncologist, and plastic surgeon. Your surgical oncologist spearheads and sets the tone for your treatment. How you feel and look after all is said and done is directly linked to them.

We have the God-given right to look and feel normal—and, dare I say, even beautiful.

This is exactly how Hoda Kotb, cohost of NBC's *Today Show*'s fourth hour (the best hour!!!) felt when she was diagnosed with breast cancer. Hoda opted to have a TRAM flap reconstruction, where the breast is re-created using the flap of skin, fat, and underlying abdominal muscle. Today, there are more than a dozen different types of flap reconstructions. But when Hoda was diagnosed in 2007, flaps were relatively new. This made her decision about her medical team even more critical. "It starts with the surgeon; at least for me it did," says Hoda. "There were so many people that were describing what they were going to do [during the surgery]. But I wanted to know what was going to be left behind when they were finished—and that does matter. So choosing the right breast cancer surgeon is important because they work in tandem with the plastic surgeon who comes in right after. It is the plastic surgeon who does most of the repair and rebuilding and how they did it mattered to me. I wanted to feel confident and comfortable."

I felt the exactly the same way. While I wasn't a candidate for any of the flap procedures, I wanted to make sure I would get a good aesthetic result. What woman doesn't want that? And by the way, we shouldn't be made to feel vain or bad about that either.

We have the God-given right to look and feel normal—and, dare I say, even beautiful.

After my diagnosis, I immediately started emailing everybody I thought would point me in the right direction. Besides my family and friends, I reached out to colleagues who wrote for health magazines, people who were connected to cancer in one way or another, and I started researching the web. After two weeks, I had a list of only three names. I made consultation appointments with each surgical oncologist to—essentially—interview them. This is what you need to do if you want to find the best possible surgeon. You wouldn't buy a car without researching its safety rating, consumer feedback, or the features it comes with. So why wouldn't you do the exact same thing when selecting your medical team? Choosing a surgeon is a life-altering decision, so it's critical to take the time to do it thoroughly.

By the last interview, I knew the questions to ask but what I was looking for was something deeper, more instinctive. "At the point where you have three doctors telling you you need a mastectomy, then you start looking for somebody who you feel like you have a connection with," says Hoda. The minute I met Dr. Elisa Port, the chief of breast surgery at Mount Sinai and the codirector of the Dubin Breast Center—I felt that connection. Dr. Port is one of the leading breast surgeons in the United States. While her qualifications are beyond impressive, she was authentically concerned for my well-being: She was kind, supportive, and provided me with all the intel I needed to make the right decision for myself. But beyond that, she never judged me for any concerns or questions I had. This became more important than her résumé when halfway through my treatment I decided not to do radiation but to have a mastectomy instead. At this point, I was in full-on panic mode—so much so that it rendered me incapable of making a decision. During one of the many visits I made to her office to discuss my options, she turned to me and said, "Sweetie, you just have to make a decision. It's going to be okay. Whatever you decide, it's going to be the right decision." She essentially gave me permission to feel good about what I wanted to do but was too scared to actually do. As I went into surgery a week later, she held my hand until I fell asleep. I will never forget her tender acts of kindness. It is those little things that make all the difference in the care you receive. For this book, I thought there would be no better authority than Dr. Port to give advice on how to find the best surgeon and what to expect from surgery. Below, she weighs in.

how to find the best *surgeon* and medical team

reputation is everything

"Number one: Look at the reputation of the medical center," advises Dr. Elisa Port, author of *The New Generation Breast Cancer Book: How to Navigate Your Diagnosis and Treatment Options—and Remain Optimistic—in an Age of Information Overload.* "You'll up your odds of getting the best possible outcome when you go to a top-tier academic center."

get recommendations

Word of mouth is very telling about the level of skill, experience, and bedside manner that you need to know when selecting your medical team. A surgeon could have extensive expertise but if they are gruff and always rushed, they may not be the best pick. When facing complicated surgeries and treatments, you will want, no, *need*, a doctor who is not only experienced but also emotionally supportive and patient with you. Cancer doesn't just take a physical toll on the body—it takes an emotional toll as well. The best way to arm yourself for the battle is to come to the field with the sharpest weapon of defense: a great surgeon. The NHS provides you with a team of specialists who work together to provide the best treatment and care. If however you are private, it is important that you choose the best surgeon for you.

look for a surgeon who specializes in your type of cancer

This rule applies for every type of cancer. If you have breast cancer, then you should look for a surgeon whose practice focuses on breast cancer surgery. If you needed brain surgery, you wouldn't go to a podiatrist, would you? No, you wouldn't. Same philosophy applies here. Dr. Port also advises looking for surgeons who have completed a fellowship within their focused cancer category. Surgeons who have completed a fellowship have dedicated an additional year beyond general surgery residency learning the latest information and the most advanced surgical techniques. "There is so much new information and things are constantly changing, developing, and progressing so rapidly," says Dr. Port. "So, you really want doctors who are very specialized and up-to-date."

inquire about the numbers

A surgeon may do breast cancer surgery but that doesn't mean they are a breast cancer surgeon. There is a *huge* difference. "The most recent statistics show that approximately 75 percent of breast cancer surgeries are performed by surgeons who do fewer than sixteen breast operations a year," reveals Dr. Port. "That's one a month. I'm doing ten to fifteen a week." This is a staggering fact that can come with serious ramifications to the patient. She adds, "There is clear-cut data demonstrating that surgeons and centers that do a high volume of specific types of surgery have better outcomes. Practice makes perfect." Don't be afraid to ask potential surgeons how many lumpectomies and mastectomies they have done every week or month. Those that hesitate to discuss their numbers are generally those who don't have an impressive number to share.

be willing to travel

Most of us are thrilled when we can hop on a plane and fly to a vacation spot. And many of us are willing to log long hours in a train or car for business. So why is it that so many people refuse to travel for health care? I understand that financial constraints and work-life obligations can make it difficult. I also know that all of us would feel more comfortable and content if our doctors were in close proximity to our homes. But that isn't always going to be the case. Traveling to a specialist who can get you healthy again is worth being out of your comfort zones—financially and physically. When my stepmother's cancer returned for the third time, my parents boarded a plane from Florida and lived temporarily in New York so she could have surgery at Memorial Sloan Kettering. After her surgeries were done, she was understandably anxious to get back home. Her New York surgeon was willing to work with a medical oncologist in Florida to oversee her chemotherapy treatments so she could recoup at home. If you can or need to travel for the best care, do it! Most doctors want you to be content and comfortable during treatment and will work on your behalf to get you home as quickly as possible.

The caveat here is that traveling to see a doctor can be expensive. Lodging, even more so, especially if longer treatment is required. Here are some organizations that can offer help:

Travel assistance

* **British Red Cross** can provide personal transport services across the UK. This includes providing a companion for a journey on public transport, or a private car with a driver. A contribution towards the cost is usually asked for, but no one will be refused a service if they can't pay. Call 0344 871 11 11 or visit www.redcross.org.uk/What-we-do/Health-and-social-care/Independent-living/Transport-support.

* **St John Wales** can provide transport for people who have difficulty using public transport or their own vehicle. Call 0292 044 9600 or visit www.stjohnwales.co.uk.

* **Tenovus Cancer Care and Mobile Support Units** specialise in chemotherapy and a mobile Lymphoedema clinic. People can be treated in their own communities, saving them long and expensive journeys to hospital. Visit www.tenovuscancercare.org.uk.

* **Air Care Alliance** offers a central listing of free transportation services provided by volunteer pilots and charitable aviation groups. Call 888-260-9707 or visit www.aircareall.org.

* **Angel Airline Samaritans** facilitates no-cost or reduced-rate commercial airline tickets to and from distant specialized medical evaluations or treatments for people with cancer in need and their families. Call 800-296-1217 or visit www.angelairlinesamaritans.org.

* **The Corporate Angel Network** arranges free air transportation for people with cancer traveling to treatment using empty seats on corporate jets. Call 866-328-1313 or visit www.corpangelnetwork.org.

* **LifeLine Pilots** are volunteer pilots who donate their time and all flight expenses to people in need of free transportation for ongoing treatment, diagnosis, and follow-up care. Call 800-822-7972 or visit www.lifelinepilots.org.

* **PALS (Patient AirLift Services)** has a network of volunteer pilots who provide people with chronic illnesses air transport services at no cost. Call 888-818-1231 or visit www.palservices.org.

Housing assistance

* **National Health Service** often offers hotel rooms near the hospital if you cannot travel for clinical tests or treatments.

* **Cotton Rooms** is a free boutique hotel for UCLH patients. You must be 'referred' by your service. Check if your NHS hospital has an equivalent. Visit cottonrooms.com.

* **Healthcare Hospitality Network** is an association of more than two hundred nonprofit organizations that provide lodging and support services to families and their loved ones who are receiving medical treatment away from home. Call 800-542-9730 or visit www.hhnetwork.org.

* **Ronald McDonald House Charities** offer free or reduced-cost lodging for families of seriously ill children who are receiving treatment at nearby hospitals. Call 630-623-7078 or visit rmhc.org.

always get a second opinion

Don't you like having options? I do! And for that reason alone I am a big advocate of getting a second opinion. It is important to know that there are some doctors—not all—who will advise a patient to do a certain type of surgery or reconstruction based on what they feel comfortable doing, and not what's in the best interest of the patient. There have been instances where patients were talked out of the type of surgery or reconstruction they wanted because it wasn't what the surgeon wanted to do. This happens more when it comes to some of the trickier or newer reconstruction surgeries, like flap reconstructions, that require time and a certain skill set that not all doctors are equipped with. If one doctor tells you not to consider a particular course of action but can't give you a reason why, that should raise some red flags. But if you talk to a few doctors and they all agree, it makes the intel more believable.

take notes

Dr. Port says it best: "This is a time of information overload." Nowhere will you feel this more strongly than the first visit, post-diagnosis, with the oncologist. Trust me when I say, it's like a crash course in Math 55 with stats, studies, and test results whizzing past your ears. If you're like me, you'll probably only absorb a third of it. And I'm not alone in that. "In the beginning, I started taking notes because there was just so much information flying at me," says Joan Lunden, who created the Internet channel ALIVE with Joan after she was diagnosed with breast cancer. "I wrote down all the questions, then I started writing down all my emotions and fears. Eventually, that's what became *Had I Known* [her *New York Times*–best-selling memoir]." Notes will help you review all the information when your mind is swimming and emotions are swirling. If writing all the information down is too emotionally draining for you, bring someone who will take notes on your behalf.

follow your gut

You may have scored a coveted appointment with one of the leading surgeons in the world but if the two of you don't click and it doesn't feel right, then follow your gut and find another surgeon. We can agree that skill and expertise rank high on the list of important qualifications, but so does getting information, time, and support. You are going to be in a long-term relationship with whatever doctor you choose, so choose one who makes you feel safe and supported.

Once you line up your medical team, then you can start thinking about surgery and treatment. For some of you, the type of cancer you have will determine what surgery and treatment you require. For others, there will be more options. Many factors come into play when making a decision, from the size of the tumor to the type of cancer, to your lifestyle, et cetera. Just know—there is not one right road to travel.

In this book, I am not going to get into the different surgeries and treatment options. I think that is better left for you to discuss with your medical team. This book is strictly a beauty guide to help you manage and care for your body as it is changing because of cancer. That said, I have had both a lumpectomy and a mastectomy, so I want to share some of the pros and cons of each, since I have lived through both experiences and know the aesthetic results you can expect.

lumpectomy
PROs:

* Minimally invasive, outpatient surgery. "I had one patient who wanted to put her kids on the school bus in the morning, have her surgery and be home in time to get them off the bus that afternoon and we made that happen," says Dr. Port.

* The incision leaves a small scar that surgeons have done wonders to minimize, often hiding along the rim of the areola.

* Quick recovery—a few days of pain and swelling (often controlled by ibuprofen) and no exercise.

* Same survival rate as mastectomy.

CONs:

* Chance of not getting clean margins. "In about 10 to 20 percent of cases we have a situation where we don't get clear margins around the tumor and we have to go in a second or third time," says Dr. Port. "That's something that a lot of people don't know about lumpectomy surgery. When you go in a second and third time and you're chiseling out more tissue, that's when you can start getting into more disfigurement."

* Unclear margins require repeat trips to the OR and, ultimately, lead to a mastectomy. "That initial incision for the lumpectomy can have huge ramifications for the patient in terms of aesthetic results if you end up needing to have mastectomy soon after," says Dr. Port. (This is just *another* reason why it's important to have an experienced surgeon who is always thinking ten steps ahead and is prepared for all possible scenarios that can play out.)

* Slightly higher chance of local recurrence after a lumpectomy versus a mastectomy.

* Radiation treatment generally consists of six weeks of daily treatments. The initial visit, where the radiation oncologist tattoos the breast, can be up to two hours. After that, daily appointments last a mere five to ten minutes. Even still, the energy of getting to the hospital or facility, waiting, undressing, having treatment, then heading home or to work—for thirty days in a row—is emotionally and physically exhausting. Some of my cancer buddies who had radiation felt that it was more grueling on their body than chemo. Something to consider.

* A breast previously radiated cannot safely tolerate additional radiation if there is a recurrence.

* The side effects of radiation are no joke. Temporary side effects include exhaustion, lymphedema, and skin burning, peeling, and discoloration—just to name a few. But it's the long-term effects that concerned me most. Radiation can cause the breast tissue to lose its elasticity and harden. "During the six weeks of radiation, there is an accumulation of injury," says my talented plastic surgeon, Dr. Leo Keegan, the medical director of Fifth Avenue Millennium Aesthetic Surgery and the assistant clinical professor of surgery, Division of Plastic Surgery, at the Icahn School of Medicine at Mount Sinai. "That injury leads to a fibrosis of all the tissue that has been radiated. You can think about it like scarring on a more cellular level. The skin, breast, and muscle will experience permanent changes where the breast tissue feels more indurated and firm leaving them not as pliable than nonradiated tissue. In implant-based reconstructions, it also creates the increased risk of capsular contracture, infection, and increased wound healing risks." This can change the appearance of the breast to the point where it appears higher, firmer, and indented at the surgical site. That hardened tissue can make it more challenging—and in some rare cases, impossible—to operate on or reconstruct. A woman I know experienced this firsthand. She had gotten breast cancer and opted to have a lumpectomy and radiation. About six years later, and a year after she finished her course of Tamoxifen, she got cancer in her other breast. When they couldn't get clear margins, she opted to have a bilateral mastectomy. In her breast that had been previously radiated, the reconstruction didn't take. Her skin lacked the elasticity it required to keep the incision closed so her expander could stretch the skin and make room for the implant. The incision kept opening, leaving her expander exposed. Her plastic surgeon had to reoperate to remove the expander. She was forced to

wait several months to allow the wound to heal. Two tries later, they were finally able to finish her reconstruction. You can only imagine how devastating this was emotionally, physically—and, let's face it—aesthetically.

mastectomy
PROs:

* If you decide from the get-go that you want to have a mastectomy, surgeons can place the incisions in such a way that scars are almost undetectable later on.

* In the right scenarios, surgeons can also perform nipple-sparing mastectomies, where a woman's nipples can be preserved. Angelina Jolie opted to have this done. While this is a technically challenging surgery, it preserves the look of a "normal," healthy breast.

* Limited follow-up screenings.

CONs:

* Permanent removal of the natural breast tissue.

* Intense surgery that requires a two- or three-day hospital stay.

* Recovery takes two to three weeks and includes dealing with surgical drains, pain meds, no exercise—among other things. For some of the flap-based reconstructions, this can extend up to six weeks.

* Depending on the type of reconstruction you decide to have, it can mean multiple surgeries. Flap reconstructions are more intense and have a longer recovery period, but all the surgery is done in one shot. With implant-based surgeries, there will be at least three surgeries including: 1) Putting in the tissue expanders—typically

done at the same time as the mastectomy—but not always. In some cases, patients can go directly to implants, avoiding the tissue expander step; 2) swapping out the expanders and replacing them with the implants; and 3) nipple reconstruction.

* Implant-based mastectomies will require at least one future "swap" surgery to replace the implants once they start to show signs of age and/or wear and tear.

* Implants can become encapsulated or rippled and they can rotate or drop—all requiring follow-up surgery to fix the issue.

* Since the breast tissue has been removed, the implant is placed under the pectoral muscle to help protect the implant. Because of this, any time the muscle is activated—like opening a jar of pickles, doing a pull-up, even if you get cold and start to shiver—it can cause the implant to move or get squeezed into a weird position temporarily. I won't lie—this looks as awkward as it sounds.

note: I understand there are some of you who will opt out of reconstruction. For those of you who do, turn to Chapter 8 (page 212) for all the intel and tips you will need about shopping for and wearing breast and nipple prostheses.

implant options

If you are considering an implant-based reconstruction, which is what I have, then you are going to have to consider the type of implant you prefer. There are three main types and each provides a different look. Below is a quick breakdown of each:

saline implants

Saline implants are much like tissue expanders because they are filled with salt water. Many patients prefer saline because they believe them to be safer; however, you should be aware that this type of implant tends to fatigue faster than silicone implants. While all implants wrinkle over time, saline implants are more likely to show visible signs of rippling and don't feel as natural as silicone. After all breast tissue is removed during a mastectomy, the only thing left cushioning the implant is the thin pectoral muscle; the round shape and ripples can be very obvious. In terms of how they feel: The salt water provides a bouncy water balloon–like touch.

silicone implants

The reason a lot of women gravitate to implants filled with liquid silicone gel is they look and feel the most natural. When you are standing, the gel rests at the bottom of the implant and assumes a teardrop shape, mimicking what the natural breast tissue does. When lying down, the fluid spreads out and tends to rest near the armpit and outer breast, again, just like normal breasts. They also feel pillowy soft. In 2010, the study "Measuring and Managing Patient Expectations for Breast Reconstruction: Impact on Quality of Life and Patient Satisfaction" revealed "patients that receive silicone breast implants reported significantly higher satisfaction with the results of reconstruction than those who had received saline implants."

cohesive silicone gel implants

In 2012, two years after the study mentioned above, teardrop-shaped cohesive silicone gel breast implants became available in the United States. These implants, which have been available in Europe for many years, are filled with a form-stable cohesive silicone. If you were to cut the implant in half, the interior gel would resemble the texture of the inside of a gummy bear. The silicone doesn't move and won't spill out. Hence its nickname "gummy bear" implants. With a thicker composition, these implants tend to ripple less than any of the other options. They also have a textured coating, which gives the implant a suedelike feel and helps prevent capsular contracture and implant rotation. Implant rotation can happen with round implants but most women don't even know it has occurred because it doesn't change the look of the breast. However, when a shaped implant rotates, it can make the breast look asymmetrical. The only fix for this is corrective surgery. So, while there are many benefits to cohesive gel implants, there are still things to keep in mind when or if you choose them.

safety concerns

There are many women who fear getting silicone breast implants. It is a fair concern. Any time you put something foreign into your body, your body can react to it. In the 1990s, many women believed their implants were causing a host of medical issues including rheumatoid arthritis, lupus, and cancer. Because of this, the FDA imposed a ban on all silicone implants until investigations could determine— one way or another –the status of their safety. In 2006, after fourteen years, the FDA lifted the ban, stating that the evidence did not link implants to subsequent health issues.

I think cancer is already a scary, emotional journey. I would caution all of you to avoid falling into the trap of letting rumor and innuendo affect your medical decisions. This goes for anything soapbox preachers will throw at you: from telling you to use all organic skin care products to what reconstruction option to choose. My advice: Quiet the background noise and focus on the facts. If you are concerned about the safety of implants, then you should read the literature, look at the FDA's findings, and discuss it with your doctors. This way, you will make an informed choice and will prevent any fear and paranoia from creeping into your thoughts later on.

I will end this discussion by sharing that my silicone implants did more than make me look and feel "normal" again. They restored my ability to feel sexy and be comfortable while intimate with my partner. Trust me when I say this isn't a given after cancer—it is a gift.

just-home-from-the-hospital beauty *must*

"After I got home from the hospital, I was still a mess. My sister said to me, 'We're going for a blowout!' She put me in a cab and took me to this blow-out place near my house," remembers Hoda. "When you've been in a hospital and your hair is matted and dirty, it makes you feel even worse. The first time they washed out all that bad stuff then blew it dry, it just made me so happy. It was a little painful because I was still sore but I didn't care; it felt so good." Her advice: When you get home from the hospital, make sure to book a wash 'n' blow at a salon close to home. If you are a friend wondering how you can make a loved one feel better, a blowout is always a feel-good treat after surgery! "That was one of my mandatories during recovery, getting a blowout once a week," she says of her healing beauty routine. "Never underestimate the power of a blowout!"

post–surgery care—such a drain!

Surgical drains are the worst. Right after waking up from a mastectomy—when you feel sore, groggy, and emotionally beaten to hell—you have to contend with surgical drains that look like hand grenades attached to tubes hanging from your body. Beside the obvious gross part—the excess blood and bodily fluids dripping from your body into the tubes—the drains are cumbersome and bulky. They make it difficult to sleep, walk about, and get dressed. "Everyone hates the drains but they are important for the healing process," says Dr. Keegan. "The scars, fortunately, are small but they can vary in how they heal."

The drains are a necessary evil. They are attached to clear tubes that rest under your skin near the surgical site, and help flush out the excess blood and lymphatic fluids that pool near the wound. The tubes may be held in place with a suture so they don't accidently slip out or leak. The weight from the drains is made heavier by the fluids and can tug on the skin, causing the incision site to become irritated, red, and swollen. It's important to make sure to empty the drains on schedule and keep them clean to prevent any disruption to the healing of the surgery. Make sure to:

1 **Keep the incision clean and dry.** Because you won't be able to shower or bathe while you have the drains, you can use a mixture of peroxide and water to keep the area clean. Apply with a Q-tip and gently dab away any residue. Make sure to dry the area by dabbing with a tissue to soak up any extra moisture.

2 **Dressings can keep the site germ-free.** While you have the drains, "There are a variety of dressings that can be applied with antibiotic ointments," says Dr. Keegan. "There's something called a biopatch, which has an antibiotic impregnation to help reduce the risk of infection." Your doctor or nurses should be applying these at the hospital. Also ask for some extra ones that you can bring home.

3 **Keep the drains hoisted up.** From the minute I woke up, my drains were secured to my hospital gown with safety pins. Safety pins!?! When I returned home and didn't have nurses to help me pin my drains to my clothes, I can't tell you how many time I pricked myself. And yes, even on painkillers, it hurt like hell. I suggest you borrow or buy a surgical bra that has built-in pockets for the drains or a drainage bulb holder, which is like a holster with Velcro straps that keeps the drains securely in place. The good thing about the drainage bulb holder is that it can be positioned around the chest, waist, hips, or thigh—so it works for whatever type of surgery or reconstruction that you've had. For advice and tips on shopping for drain holders and surgical bras, turn to Chapter 8 (page 196).

4 **Stay on top of your drain schedule.** If you miss emptying out your drains they will get heavy and pull on your skin. If you fidget with them too much, you will cause unnecessary irritation. You should have them for two weeks tops—so be diligent with them during this time. It will soon be over.

5 **Prevent scarring.** Once the drains are out and the incisions have fully healed, you can start treatment to prevent scarring. The how-to is listed below.

scar-tactics

how to minimize your scars

Scars are an unavoidable result of surgery. Some of you will wear them like a badge of honor. Others will want to wipe them from view and memory. I get it. Every time I look at my scars I am reminded that I am a survivor—something I'm damn proud of (and you should be, too!). But as a young, unmarried woman, I would prefer if I didn't have two red ropy trails running across my boobs. Hoda, who was newly divorced, felt the same way. "I remember the first time after surgery that I saw my scars," says Hoda. "After they cleaned me up, the nurse said, 'Just turn toward the mirror' and I looked up and was like 'Oh my God.' I was horrified. I had a hip-to-hip incision and then all the stuff they did on top. Don't get me wrong, I was grateful to be alive. But there was a part of me that thought nobody would ever see my body again."

The early days after surgery are no joke. Your body might look like a road map and you will probably feel like you were hit by a truck. As trite as this sounds, don't let this get you down. Recovery takes time. Scars—both emotional and physical—take time to heal. "After a while, there comes a point in your life where you accept the

> **Never be ashamed of a scar. It simply means you were stronger than whatever tried to hurt you.**
>
> **—UNKNOWN**

scars as the new normal," says Hoda. "You accept that this is your journey and this is a part of who you are. It shapes you, but it doesn't define you."

For those of you who want to erase all traces of your scars from existence, there are more options than ever before. So, let's start with the basics.

What is a scar? Whenever you get hurt, collagen—the most abundant, structural protein in the human body—springs into action to help you start healing. With deep injuries, like surgical wounds, your body produces collagen to help fill in the cut and heal the skin back together again. In some cases, when the body senses major trauma, like a surgical incision, it can overproduce collagen, causing the wound to get red and rise above the site. In other cases, the scar can become indented or weblike. There are many variables that will determine what your scars look like. This includes: how experienced your surgeon is; how your body heals; if there is any tension on the scar; if the scar gets irritated or infected; and how well you take care of your incisions during the healing process.

"A scar starts the moment of surgery, so the number one most important thing is to find a surgeon with a lot of experience," says leading scar specialist Dr. Jill Waibel, chief of dermatology at Baptist Hospital of Miami and founder of Miami Dermatology & Laser Institute. "Then, the postoperative care starts the minute surgery is done because that first week is really critical for healing."

In the early days, right after surgery, do *exactly* what your surgeon tells you. If they tell you not to exercise, not to lift heavy things, not to clean—just listen. Most damage and infections are caused when a patient pushes it and does something they shouldn't. Ladies—take a chill pill and just relax for these two weeks. Your healing is more important than doing the dishes or getting in a light workout. If you need help around the house, recruit some friends to pitch in. The most important thing is to care for your incisions. "You don't walk out of the OR with a bad scar," says Dr. Waibel. "That happens later in the ball game."

proper wound care

Below is all the info you will need to care for your incisions so you can heal beautifully.

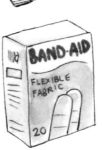

1   **Keep the incision clean:** Soak a face cloth in warm soapy water, and then gently clean the area. Pat dry with a towel, then dab on a little petroleum jelly. Be careful of antibacterial topicals creams and ointments with neomycin or bacitracin as they can cause allergic reactions.

2   **Keep it covered:** Use breathable gauze and paper tape or large Band-Aids to protect the wound. This helps shield the incision from anything rubbing up against the sutures creating friction that results in an irritation or, worse, an infection. It also shields it from airborne impurities, dirt, and germs.

3 **Hands off:** As the skin heals, your wound will get itchy—don't scratch it! Other than cleaning or applying fresh dressing, you should not touch the incision at all.

4 **Be patient:** Scars take time to heal. That's just the nature of the beast. Facial skin takes a least one week to heal. The chest and torso about two to four weeks. Legs take up to six months.

Once your sutures are removed or dissolve—seven to ten days after surgery—you should begin compression using silicone sheets like ScarAway or Steri-Strips. Compression is key because of how it affects fibroblasts, the important cells that make collagen. Essentially, the pressure of the sheets or strips alerts the fibroblast to turn off, relaying the message that the skin is finished healing. This prevents the buildup of collagen that leads to red, raised scars. "The studies haven't borne out that there's a huge improvement, but I'll tell you, having seen thousands and thousands of scar patients for the last fifteen years, you can really tell a difference when patients have done a good job with compression," says Dr. Waibel. That little extra step of applying a silicone sheet for the first three months makes a *huge* difference in the overall visual result you will end up with. And that lasts a lifetime. By the seventh month after surgery, if your scar is looking good, then you're probably in the clear. "It's kind of counterintuitive because most people are like, 'I want to heal. I want to give my body time to heal before I start wearing the sheets or lasering'—but it's quite the opposite," she says. "The sooner you start applying pressure, the sooner you start thinking of your scar, the better the scar will be."

types of scars

Here is a quick breakdown on the most common types of post-surgical scars, tips for how to conceal them or get rid of them altogether:

hypertrophic

Look and feel: These scars are usually red, raised, and contained to the actual size of the wound. These are the scars you will have after a lumpectomy, mastectomy, and/or reconstruction. They tend to fade over time.

Cover it: A creamy concealer can help smooth over the bumpy texture. One with a greenish tone will help neutralize red tones.

Remove it: Depending on the scar's thickness, you'll need two to seven injections of a corticosteroid like Kenalog or similar. You'll also want to wear silicone gel sheets (around £20 at Boots or online) that will apply light pressure to help prevent collagen from building back up. For new scars, you'll need to wear the gel sheets for eight to twelve weeks. For old scars, you'll need to wear them for three to six months. The scars will still be visible, but much less noticeable.

atrophic

Look and feel: These scars are recessed, like little skin-colored potholes. Think chicken pox or cystic acne. They can also be caused when a surgical scar pulls apart. "When the wound is under tension or if you've had an infection, that's when a white, thin, or pulled-apart scar results," says Dr. Waibel.

Cover it: Hiding recess scars used to be almost impossible. However, there are now skin-toned silicone putties that fill in divots and hide them beautifully. Dermaflage (£25, www.jdharris.co.uk) is an almost miracle worker in this regard. It comes with a primer that adheres the putty to the skin and a texture pad that helps mimic the surface of the skin. It dries in a minute and lasts up to thirty-six hours.

Remove it: Fractional ablative lasers (about £1300 per session) help vaporize the scar tissue. Afterward, an injection of Sculptra, a polylactic acid filler (about £500 for 2–5 vials), pops those divots up. While the effects of Sculptra are temporary—two years tops—it helps stimulate the growth of collagen. Generally, two to five combo treatments are needed and are not covered by the NHS.

contractured

Look and feel: Any time there is a loss of skin or tension on a wound, it can result in scars that are weblike in texture and marbleized in color. These scars are often a result from burns or reconstructions when there is a loss or lack of skin at the incision site.

Cover it: Microskin is a waterproof liquid that can be customized to precisely match your skin tone. It acts as a second skin, filling in and covering the scar. It stays on skin for several days, even through sweat and showers. The starter kit (£150, www.microskineurope.eu) lasts about a month depending on the size of your scar.

Remove it: If range of motion is an issue, physical therapy will help, while steroid injections and fractional ablative lasers (about £1300) help break up excessive collagen. These are often used in combination with Z-plasty, during which a Z-shaped incision at the site helps remove the scarred skin and muscle tension. (All four treatments are sometimes covered by the NHS.) While these scars can be minimized, unfortunately, they rarely disappear.

keloid

Look and feel: These scars tend to be reddish or purple-ish in color. They feel ropy and grow over the wound site. They can range in size from a pimple to an orange.

Cover it: An opaque concealer specifically designed for scars contains concentrated pigments that mean you don't have to layer on a ton of it. Choose one that matches your skin tone, then dab it on with a small synthetic concealer brush. Synthetic bristles won't absorb the product and can get into the hard-to-reach crevices of the skin.

Remove it: Steroid injections used to be the popular treatment for keloids; however, they often cause hyperpigmentation on dark skin. "I cut off most of the scar, then use a fractional ablative laser," says Dr. Waibel. This creates a small wound that the body then repairs like normal skin while removing overgrowth. This ten-minute procedure costs about £1000 and may be covered by the NHS.

under construction: building *nipples* from nothing

One of the reasons I decided to have a mastectomy was because I didn't want one single cancer cell remaining behind. I thought it was best to wipe the slate clean—so to speak—and get rid of everything, nipples included. After my implant swap surgery, all that remained were what I call "Barbie Boobs"—nipless mounds that look like those on the iconic blond doll.

There's really nothing weirder than a pair of breasts with no nipples. I know, because I lived without them for five months. While I was in treatment, one of my dearest friends, Carly, got engaged and asked me to be a bridesmaid. Right after my reconstruction, our group of eight bridesmaids flew to Austin, Texas, for Carly's bachelorette weekend. The day we arrived, we didn't waste any time—we pulled on our bathing suits and headed straight to the rooftop pool party. We weren't the only ones with that brilliant idea—all thirteen bachelor and bachelorette groups staying at the W Hotel were up there. While we lounged around, an assortment of single men kept checking out my boobs and offering to buy me drinks. I just kept thinking, "If they only knew I had no nipples!" Of course, I accepted the free drinks! I figured I might as well enjoy the upside of having a mastectomy: Boys liked my boobs and were willing to buy me booze. Silver linings!

Traveling with a group of girls inevitably puts you in close proximity that can lead to awkward moments. This is especially true when you are losing your hair and have no nipples. One day, the group of us went shopping and ended up huddled into one of those open-area fitting rooms. The salesperson interpreted my hesitation of taking off a top as me having literal trouble taking off the top, and without asking, came over and lifted it over my head. Until that moment, most of the women hadn't seen my Barbie Boobs. Some didn't even know the extent of my illness. But the second that top was off—all eyes were on my nipless chest. I acted fast—yelling—"Holy shit! My nipple just fell under the couch!" Carly, always quick on her feet, quickly yelled back while pointing under the couch, "It's under there, it's under there!" Nobody knew what to think or do. In shock and disbelief, each girl bent down and looked. This made Carly and me crack up until we were crying from laughter. From that moment on, whenever there was a potentially awkward situation, Carly and I would yell, "Oh my God, your nipple fell under the table!" It made some hard moments nothing short of hilarious. It became a running joke until I got nipples tattooed on.

The point being—having no nipples, which will be the case for some of you, is, to put it mildly, an incredibly surreal experience. When I would catch a glimpse of myself in the mirror and see the scarred mounds on my chest, it would leave me feeling completely unfeminine and detached from my body. By the time many of us get to the end of reconstruction, we are completely zapped, emotionally and physically. For this reason, I understand why many women opt to forgo nipple reconstruction. It's one more surgery, plus tattoos, that can extend this already lengthy journey another six months. What you choose to do is up to you. Personally, I am a big advocate for finishing *all* the phases of reconstruction. Not only do they complete the look of the breasts, but once they are done you can close the door on this difficult chapter in your life.

So let's chat about nipple reconstruction and nipple tattoos.

nipple reconstruction

This is surgery done to create or mimic the projection of a natural breast. It is conducted three or four months after the implant phase of reconstruction has had time to heal. It is an outpatient surgery done under twilight aesthetic. Working on the chest, where the nipple would be, the surgeon makes a few incisions creating a loose flap of skin from the scar. The sides of the flap are then folded together to create a mound that is then stitched in place. There are a number of different types of nipple flaps including the Alamo, star flap, skate flap, and the C-V flap—just to name a few. Each surgeon has a preference of the flap they prefer—but each generates similar results. Since reconstructed nipples lose up to 50 percent of the projection they had right after surgery, some surgeons will fill the core of the nipple to prevent it from flattening out over time. Typically, this is done with either a dermal matrix filler, like AlloDerm, or fat or scar tissues harvested from the patient's body.

After the reconstruction is complete, your doctor will place a nipple shield—a protective covering shaped like a pointed hat and brim—filled with antibacterial ointment over the site. The shield should be left on for three days—during which you cannot get it wet.

I wanted to make sure my nipples didn't flatten out so I kept mine covered for over a week. When you remove the shield, your nipple(s) will be swollen and puffy. As the swelling subsides, roughly about two weeks, the nipple will shrink back down to an average size.

Over time, nipples can flatten out entirely. A small shot of injectable filler like Restylane will provide instant projection. I highly recommended if you are going to get fillers to help your headlights that you go to your plastic surgeon, or a plastic surgeon who specializes in reconstruction, to do the injection. The last thing you need to deal with is a punctured implant. Personally, I like having projection. I think it gives reconstructed breasts a realness that can't be achieved with tattoos alone. It provides one more detail that helps restore the look and feel of being "normal" again.

nipple tattoos

These are done on breast cancer patients who were not candidates for, or who have opted against, having a nipple-sparing mastectomy. The tattoos are typically done three to five months after the nipple reconstruction has healed. Traditionally, nipple tattoos have been performed by a patient's plastic surgeon, or someone on his staff. Today, as surgical techniques advance and aesthetic results get better, more and more patients are expecting the same level of quality and realism in every area and phase of their reconstruction. This especially applies to the nipple tattoos—which can make or break the look of a reconstruction.

I was no stranger to tattoo parlors, having gotten inked my first year in college. As I got older, the ink began to fade and spread. It looked really tacky. Rather than have it covered with another design, I opted have to have it lasered off. It was a small black tattoo, so I figured it would come off quickly. Wrong. What I learned, the hard way, is tattoo removal is a lengthy, painful, expensive process. My little tat took eight appointments and cost me more than $3,000. It also removed the natural pigment of my skin, leaving behind a white halo, outlining where the tattoo had been.

That little lesson ended up serving me well. When it was time for the final phase of my reconstruction—the nipple tattoos—I approached it like I was writing an investigative news story. I spent hours researching online and questioning some of my cancer buddies. What I saw frightened me. Most of the nipple tattoos out there were really bad. Like, *really* bad. The *best* way I can describe the tattoos I saw: pepperoni slices. They were perfectly round, overly red, and had no dimension.

Here's the crux of the problem: Most nipple tattoos are performed by the plastic surgeon in charge of the reconstruction. In some (most) cases, the procedure isn't even done by the doctor but by someone on his staff. With only a few hours of tattoo training, most of these professionals don't have the skill to create a realistic nipple. They don't know how to mix pigments to create nuanced shades. They don't know how to draw shadows and highlights to create dimension. They can't freehand the slightly imperfect shape of an areola. The end result is usually a passing resemblance to the real thing—a one-dimensional, reddish, pink, or brown overly perfect circle inked on the breast. It's no wonder there are so many bad nipple tattoos out there.

Let me be clear: I have the highest regard for surgeons and their staff, but I wouldn't go to a tattoo artist to perform a mastectomy, so why would I go to a plastic surgeon to give me a tattoo? It makes no sense. Getting the best result all comes back to finding the most skilled person trained to do the job. This is true of your surgeon, your oncologist—even down to your tattoo artist.

I decided I wouldn't get my nipples done until I found a trained tattoo artist who could create the look I wanted. A few days later, I came across a survivor's blog with a small post about her new 3-D nipple tattoos. If I hadn't read the post, I would have believed her nipples were the real deal. But when I read that a tattoo artist named

tit-tillating tidbit

In 1977, an exotic dancer living in the Mission District of San Francisco popped into her local beauty boutique looking for a makeup product that she could use to make her nipples appear rosier and perkier. The product, she explained, had to be long lasting, as it needed to stay on through her dance routines. The two shop owners didn't sell anything like it but promised the dancer something by the next day. That night, they went home and whipped up a cherry-hued stain from steaming fresh rose petals. That shop was the first of many for Benefit Cosmetics. And that stain, now called Benetint, has gone on to become a cult-favorite cheek and lip stain among celebrities and makeup artists. In fact, one Benetint is sold every two minutes, making it one of the top-selling makeup products of all time.

Today, the stain has come full circle and is used as a popular beauty hack for breast cancer patients. During the time between surgery and nipple reconstruction when you have nothing but "Barbie Boobs" (breast mounds without nipples), applying Benetint to the center of the breasts will help you fake the effect of real areolas. Whether you want to create a shadowy effect under a light blouse or to make your breasts look "normal" while being intimate with your partner, the flushed stain will help give you a rosier perspective in life.

Vinnie Myers had inked her realistic nipples, my jaw dropped. I Googled his name and found his website. Once there, I spent hours looking through one tattoo after the next—and all of them looked totally believable. I called right then and booked an appointment at Little Vinnie's Tattoos in Finksburg, Maryland. The earliest slot was five months away.

Vinnie Myers is a former army medic, who learned to tattoo by inking his military buddies while on duty. For years, he perfected his craft creating intricate and colorful sleeves and back pieces. Then, one fateful night at a party, he struck up a conversation with a woman who worked for a plastic surgeon. She explained that they were having a difficult time tattooing their breast cancer patients and asked if he would mind coming in to help correct some of the tattoos they had done. After a few jobs, Vinnie quickly recognized the need for trained tattoo artists to be involved in breast reconstruction. Just as quickly, word got out in the breast cancer community about the realistic tattoos he was creating. Pretty soon, women from as far away as Dubai were flying to the United States to get their "Vinnies." His 3-D nipple tattoos have earned him the nickname, "the Michelangelo of Nipple Tattoos."

"I get to see tattoos done by different doctors from all over the world and it never ceases to amaze me how bad most of them are," says Vinnie. "I've seen tattoos that don't match a woman's skin tone or her existing areola, nipples that are so large and out of proportion they take up half the breast, or nipples that are positioned so far on the sides they are almost in the armpits."

Vinnie's work is quite the opposite. He creates symmetrical nipples in hues that match the unique coloring of each woman that stands before him. But the devil is in the details. Vinnie's 3-D details go so far to include the Montgomery glands—the little glands that secrete oil that help with breastfeeding. "All I'm doing is creating the image of these little bumps with a highlight and a shadow," says Vinnie. "It's art 101—highlights and shadows give you the illusion of dimension. But it's something that most doctors don't know how to do."

When I first walked into Little Vinnie's, I had Barbie Boobs. When I left I had beautiful breasts. But the best part was that when I walked out of his tattoo parlor, I walked into the next phase of my life with some perky porn-star boobies leading the way…

how to find a nipple tattoo artist

Because I had such a difficult time trying to find someone who could create realistic nipple tattoos, I figured this must be the case for most breast cancer survivors. I decided to chronicle this last phase of my reconstruction by writing about it for the *New York Times*, in a piece titled "A Tattoo That Completes a New Breast." A video, created by the *New York Times*'s talented video editor, Kassie Bracken, accompanied the piece. When the story was published, it went viral with more than ten million views.

To me, this signifies the overwhelming need and desire for talented tattoo artists like Vinnie Myers to be involved in reconstructions and provide this life-changing service. It is my hope that in the near future plastic surgeons will take part in this dialogue and begin working with trained tattoo artists to achieve the best reconstruction results possible. Healthcare—in any aspect—should always be about the benefit to the patient over the potential for profit.

So what should you do if you want a tattoo but can't see Vinnie? I posed this question to the man himself and here are his tips for finding a skilled tattoo artist:

* **Experience matters.** "It is extremely important to go to a tattoo artist who has experience working on reconstructed breasts," says Vinnie. "Postoperative anatomy is very different than working on a normal breast. The skin is thinner, the breast tissue is gone, the pectoral muscle is stretched paper-thin, and then you have the implant. But a regular tattoo artist isn't going to know that. If they tattoo at a normal tattoo depth, they will tattoo the muscle or puncture the implant—and that will cause damage to the reconstruction and the woman's health. An experienced artist will be able to tell the integrity of the skin and tissue and keep you and your reconstruction safe."

* **Pictures please!** You've heard the expression, "A picture is worth a thousand words." Well, in this case, it is worth so much more. Pictures are a direct indicator of what your tattoo will look like. "Once you find an artist that has done nipple tattoos, ask to see the photographs of the tattoos they've done and see what the quality of those tattoos looks like," says Vinnie. "If you were going to have a regular tattoo done, you'd look at an artist's portfolio before getting a tat from them. It's the same deal. If they don't have any pictures or the pictures don't look good, don't get the tattoo from them."

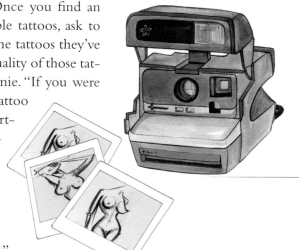

* **Ask the important questions.** "Tattoo artists aren't known to be the friendliest people," warns Vinnie. Conversations, especially those centered around nipples, might prove a little uncomfortable. That said, persevere. "It's crucial to ask as many questions as possible," he says. "Ask, 'How many nipple tattoos have you done?' 'Are you familiar with tattooing over an implant?' 'Do you know what a TRAM flap is?' 'Do you know what a DIEP flap is?'" The answers to your questions will be telling in how much they know and how experienced they are.

* **Talk to other survivors.** Pictures don't lie but, sadly, people do. There have been cases where tattoo artists have stolen images of other artists' work and passed it off as their own. It is important to protect yourself against such deception. Cancer patients tend to be more vulnerable, because they can allow hope to override

common sense. Ask the tattoo artist if you can speak to some of his clients who have gotten nipple tattoos. If they aren't willing to make the connection, you have to ask yourself why. Word-of-mouth recommendations will help point you in the right direction every time.

* **Do your research.** "There are trained professionals all over that do nipple tattoos," says Vinnie. "There is a website called the pinkink project.com with an unvetted list of tattooers. It will be your job to sort through the list and determine the quality of work each artist is doing. But at least it's a place to start." If you are having a hard time finding a tattoo artist online, you can also try searching the following titles: cosmetic tattoo artist, permanent makeup artists, paramedical tattoo specialists, and micropigmentation specialists. Once you find one of these professionals, make sure to look at their portfolio and speak to some of their clients. Fancy titles don't always translate into fancy artwork.

* **Know the cost.** Nipple tattoos range in cost depending on the professional you are getting them from. Some NHS hospitals cover the cost. Some paramedical or cosmetic tattooers charge upward of £5000, and, if private, some insurances will cover part of the cost. Tattoo artists, like Vinnie, charge around £300 to £700. My insurance would not reimburse the cost, even though I got a patient advocate and tried to arbitrate. Ultimately, I ended up covering the cost out of pocket.

* **Be willing to wait.** I hate to state the obvious, but a tattoo is permanent. Once it's done—it's hard to undo. This is especially true when working on compromised, delicate skin. Vinnie says, "It is better to wait two years to get the good tattoo, then to get a horrible tattoo quickly that takes two years to correct—and that ruins your reconstruction in the process."

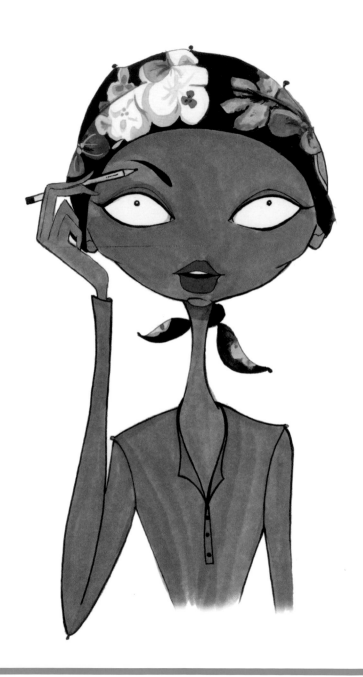

CHAPTER 7

MAKEUP IS THE BEST MEDICINE

how color is curative

I wasn't always a glamour girl. To be honest, it feels odd even referring to myself as such. I am much happier when I can leave the house with a bare face and a quick swipe of lip gloss. For most of my life, wearing makeup was like owning a dog I couldn't train. I loved it to death, but I didn't know what the hell I was doing and I had no control over it. Don't get me wrong, I've always loved playing with makeup. But most of the time I ended up looking like a hot mess rather than looking hot. It wasn't until I left my job as a newspaper fashion columnist to be a magazine beauty editor that things started to change. As part of my new job, I got to interview the leading makeup artists in the beauty industry. They shared their tips and tricks and I started trying them at home. In just a few years, I had transformed into a full-fledged beauty junkie who knew how to contour better than the Kardashians. But just as I was at the top of my glamour game, I was diagnosed with cancer.

I think beauty is elusive for most of us. One day we look awesome, the next day, not so much. Trying to look good on the regular is a roller coaster. It gets even trickier when you are in treatment. By the time I was diagnosed my entire world centered around beauty. During the appointment when my oncologist told me I would have to have chemo, I remember thinking "How am I going to do my job as a beauty editor with green skin, patchy lashes, and no eyebrows?" My health and career were on a collision course. But here's the thing: When your whole world is shifting, there are few things that remain constant. When my body started changing and I felt like I was losing myself, the staples in my makeup bag—my Sara Happ lip gloss, Bobbi Brown eyeliner, and RMS blush—reminded me of the girl I was before cancer and the woman I wanted to be after it. Lipsticks *are* lifesavers. One swipe reminds you that there is life to be lived and you should show up for it! So, when you find yourself too tired, too sad, too sick—my advice is to keep the glam going. It doesn't have to be a full face of makeup. A subtle swirl of blush is all you need to lift your cheeks and your mood. Trust me on this.

Two nights after I was diagnosed, I went out to dinner with my dear friend Ramy Gafni. Ramy created a name for himself as the brow guru of Hollywood. If there's a pair of A-list arches you envy, chances are Ramy has worked his magic on them. He is also an amazing makeup artist to boot. Not a bad friend to have—I'll tell you that! Ramy and I became friends through work but our bond became stronger when I was diagnosed with cancer. Ramy is also a cancer survivor. He was diagnosed with non-Hodgkin's lymphoma right before his thirty-second birthday and started chemo the day after. During his battle, he wrote his first book, *Ramy Gafni's Beauty Therapy: The Ultimate Guide to Looking and Feeling Great While Living with Cancer.*

> *I'm not saying that putting on makeup will change the world or even your life, but it can be a first step in learning things about yourself you may never have discovered otherwise. At worst, you could make a big mess and have a good laugh.*
>
> **—ICONIC MAKEUP ARTIST KEVYN AUCOIN (1962–2002), *FACE FORWARD***

When I was diagnosed, Ramy's words of encouragement and his stellar makeup advice helped me look like my old self. For thirteen years, Ramy gave free makeup lessons at Cancer Care, a national organization that provides services to those affected by the disease. As a beauty director I have always known how powerful makeup can be, but with Ramy's help I discovered that cosmetics are also curative. "It's not about looking like Cindy Crawford," he says. "It's about looking like yourself before you started treatment."

But Ramy isn't the only makeup artist who came, brush in hand, to help me out. Sonia Kashuk, the celeb makeup artist whose name-sake line is a best seller at Target, was there for me from day one. As a stage I breast cancer survivor, Sonia got me in to see her surgical oncologist, Dr. Elisa Port. She was vital to me in the early days when

I felt paralyzed by fear, ignorance, and the information overload that comes with a cancer diagnosis. She picked up the phone more than once to offer her guidance, love, and support. I was a huge fan of her line before the cancer, but now I am an even bigger fan of the woman behind it. While she is wildly busy and successful, she continues to be generous with her time and energy, especially for those affected by this shitty disease. Among her many titles, she is the spokesperson for Cancer and Careers. "I love the work that I've done over the years but the most rewarding thing on a personal level is giving back to women and trying to help them with this difficult journey," says Sonia. "There is light at the end of the tunnel."

Like Ramy, Sonia's been around this cancer block and knows a thing or two about how to offset the visual side effects of treatment. Their advice comes from having lived it. Below are their makeup tips that will have you looking gorg in no time!

tip: try, then buy!

When you're going through treatment, your makeup routine is going to be trial and error. Certain makeup brands, formulations, and shades that worked for you before, might not work now. "Keep an open mind," says Ramy. "And treat yourself a little bit. It's okay to buy an extra foundation to see if it's going to work on you." Most drugstores and some department stores will allow you to return or exchange products if they aren't flattering or if you don't like the formula. If the store gives you a hassle, this is where I give you permission to use your cancer card. You shouldn't have to spend a lot of money to look or feel good. "Ask for samples," he advises. "This way you can test a product to see if the color is a good match or if it irritates your skin before buying it. You might also discover a new product you love at the same time!"

makeup for "*mood skin*"

You've all heard of mood rings, right? Made with thermotropic crystals, these rings change color based on body temperature and can, supposedly, tell the mood of the wearer. Well, get ready—'cause during treatment, your skin tone will most likely change just like a mood ring. This is something a lot of patients don't expect. "I had what I like to call 'mood skin,'" says Ramy. "One day it was gray, the next day it was yellow, the next day it was white, the next day it was green."

It can be a challenge on an average day to find makeup—especially foundations and concealers—that flatter your individual skin tone perfectly. Add mood skin into the mix and it becomes a daunting task. Techniques, the way you should apply your makeup, are also tricky. Below is a list of products and application tips that will help.

getting a primer

Tip: Less is more when it comes to makeup during cancer. When we can scale back on products and steps, our routines get easier and we look healthier for it. That said, there will be times when your skin is misbehaving and you may need or want to call in reinforcements to help deal with it. During my chemo, I broke out in hives and got acne. Not only was it physically uncomfortable, it made me feel self-conscious. I followed doctor's orders by taking Benadryl and using cortisone cream but I needed a faster fix so I could put my best face forward at work. That product was a silicone-based makeup primer. "When your skin texture is changing or if you have any discoloration, primers help make the surface of the skin smoother and even toned," says Ramy. "They also provide grip so your makeup looks fresher, longer."

Try: Japonesque Velvet Touch Primer, Maybelline Baby Skin Instant Pore Eraser, Smashbox Photo Finish Foundation Primer, and NYX Studio Perfect Primer.

Technique: After washing your face, dab it dry, then apply moisturizer and sunblock. Allow them to absorb into the skin, then apply a primer. Those formulated specifically for long-wear *really* stay put. I use my fingertips to apply in a circular motion, giving myself a mini facial massage to get the blood flowing at the same time. I apply primer all over my face when I have a meeting or am going out. On casual days, I spot-apply only using a small brush just to zhuzh under and around my eyes. Either way, a little goes a long way—and the results are worthy of a selfie.

cover up!

Tip: Concealer is the makeup equivalent of a perfect pair of jeans. For starters, it's a staple that you can build the rest of your look around. It also has the ability to transform your skin and features in ways you never imagined. Whether you want to erase shadowy under-eye circles, spot-cover a blemish, or help sculpt your cheekbones— concealer is the product that does the trick. Basically, it allows you to be the best version of yourself. Who's not down for that?

Try: Clé de Peau Beauté Concealer, Kevyn Aucoin The Sensual Skin Enhancer, Revlon PhotoReady Concealer, and CoverGirl truBLEND FIXSTICK Concealer. My all-time favorite is Cinema Secrets Ultimate Corrector 5-in-1 Pro Palette, which has five shades of creamy concealer so you can customize the color as your skin changes from season to season or, in this case, when you have mood skin.

Technique: "Concealer that is very pigmented and blendable is very important," says Ramy. "Opt for one with yellow undertones, which neutralizes redness and is the best at covering dark spots." Color-correcting concealers are also an option. They come in three shades— lilac, yellow, and green. Each color neutralizes problematic undertones in the skin. Green nixes red or ruddy tones like a blemish or a port wine stain. Yellow erases brown tones like sun or age spots. Lilac hides hyperpigmentation.

I generally prefer stick concealers because they stay put longer. But regardless of the type you prefer, make sure it is creamy and moisturizing. Sticks tend to be waxier and stiffer, so just make sure to test it out before buying or using. You want one that glides on easily and won't require too much rubbing to blend it into the skin. Apply a small dot just on the area you want to cover, then gently blend out to the surrounding area. I like using my finger because my body heat warms the concealer and makes it easier to blend. If you prefer a brush, use one with synthetic bristles and a dome or slightly pointed tip. These are the best for covering the small nooks of the face like the inner corner of the eye and around the edge of the nostril. A mini sponge (like the baby BeautyBlender) will soak up more product and isn't the most precise but is great for creating a diffused, airbrushed effect. Also, apply concealer before base makeup. Most of us don't need as much foundation when our imperfections are hidden.

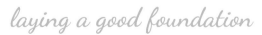

laying a good foundation

Tip: Even if you're not used to wearing a foundationlike product, now might be the time to try one. The good news is there are more options than ever before. They come in a mix of textures and formulas, upping the chances that you will find one that's a perfect match.

Below is a quick breakdown of the different types of base makeup that can help even out the natural tone of your skin and—dare we say—make it appear flawless.

tinted moisturizer

The name is self-explanatory. The product gives you a hint of sheer color with a moisturizing benefit.

Try: Laura Mercier Tinted Moisturizer, La Mer The Reparative Skin-Tint Broad Spectrum SPF 30, Stila Sheer Color Tinted Moisturizer SPF 20, and Neutrogena Healthy Skin Glow Sheers Illuminating Tinted Moisturizer with SPF 30.

BB cream

The Korean beauty invasion introduced us to some amazing new products—most notably beauty balms (BBs). BB creams are just like tinted moisturizers but with added skin care benefits and ingredients, including SPF and antioxidants. My only advice is don't count on them for your sun protection. Even though they contain some UVA/UVB filters, they aren't enough to do the job of traditional sunscreen, especially during treatment. They are generally sold in broad shades like light, medium, and dark.

Try: Maybelline Dream Fresh BB Cream, Bobbi Brown BB Cream, Dr. Brandt Signature Flexitone BB Cream, Garnier Skin Renew Miracle Perfector B.B. Cream, and Avon Ideal Flawless BB Beauty Balm Cream.

CC cream

Similar in concept to a BB cream, the main function of a CC is "color correcting." In terms of texture and coverage, they are the middle children: more opaque than a tinted moisturizer or BB but lighter than a foundation. They are formulated with targeted ingredients and light-reflecting particles that conceal and correct issues like redness, sallowness, and hyperpigmentation (sun or age spots).

Try: It Cosmetics Your Skin But Better CC+ Cream with SPF 50+, Peter Thomas Roth CC Cream, L'Oréal Nude Magique Anti-Redness CC Cream, and Aveeno Active Naturals Positively Radiant CC Cream SPF 30.

DD cream

Depending on whom you talk to, these balms have a few names including: "daily defense," "dermatologically defining," and "dynamic do-all." DDs have all the benefits the other alphabet creams brag about—SPF sun protection and coverage—but they up the ante with antiaging ingredients that help reduce fine lines and sun damage and smooth skin.

Try: Julep DD Créme and DERMAdoctor DD Cream.

foundation

While alphabet creams offer a lot of benefits, there are many people who still prefer using this classic cosmetic. For starters, foundations come in a range of shades and textures and can be customized to create a perfect match for your skin.

Try: Charlotte Tilbury Magic Foundation, Maybelline Fit Me! Foundation, Giorgio Armani Maestro Fusion Makeup, Benefit Hello Flawless Foundation, and Tom Ford Traceless Foundation Stick.

Technique: Selecting the perfect shade of base makeup can be tricky. Some makeup artists suggest matching it to your wrist or along your jawline. However, if you are dealing with mood skin or have hyperpigmentation from radiation, neither of these will help you find the right foundation shade. Instead, Ramy suggests selecting one that matches the area where your cheek and under-eye area meet. This spot is where the lightest and most colorful areas of your face meet—so you score a color that works for both. "During one of my makeup classes, a survivor showed how half her face, part of her cheek and down her neck, had been burned from radiation and healed darker than the rest of her complexion," says Ramy. "Every time she went to a department store beauty counter to get help, they would match the foundation to the darker area. She said to me, 'That's not me. That's not the color I was before radiation. I was lighter.' I showed her how to match her skin with the lighter shade using a foundation stick, which tends to be more pigmented and thicker so they provide more coverage and adhere longer. Needless to say, she was beyond thrilled."

The best way to achieve even coverage is by applying the product down the center of the face (where you generally need the most coverage), then blending it outward to the edges (where you need the least). Sonia also suggests applying face oil to the skin a few minutes before foundation. "I put a little on under my eyes or any place that feels dry or looks dull," says Sonia. "I let it soak into the skin for five or six minutes and then I apply my foundation. This makes the skin look a little glowier without looking like you have a lot of product on."

tip: don't dull your shine!

"I am a big believer in skin looking slightly dewy, so I suggest staying away from powder products, like foundation and blush, because they make the skin look flat," says Sonia. "The goal is to achieve dimension, a little lift and brightness. Cream products have more of a luminous finish and leave the skin looking lit from within."

bronzer: get a healthy glow

Tip: "As far as mood skin goes, the solution is bronzer," says Ramy. "I started using bronzer every day [during treatment] and I just looked healthy." (Yes—this tip also works for men!) When choosing a bronzer, opt for one that is two shades darker than your skin, with a matte finish. Bronzers with peach or pink undertones will help offset any jaundice (yellow), waxy (white), or puke-y (green) tinges in the skin. To avoid looking like an Oompa Loompa, steer clear of formulas that are dark, shimmery, or obviously orange.

Try: Benefit Hoola Matte Bronzer, NYX Matte Bronzer, Guerlain Terracotta Sheer Bronzing Powder, Nars Bronzing Powder, and Smashbox Bronze Lights.

Technique: The trick to achieving natural sun-kissed color has a lot to do with the brush you use. The bigger the brush, the more sheer and even the application of color. To find the perfect size, look for a large fluffy brush where the dome of the bristles is a little bit bigger than the apple of your cheeks, Dip the brush into the bronzer, then swirl onto the areas of the face that would normally get the most color—forehead, nose, cheeks, and chin. Another way to achieve a healthy glow is "get a cream bronzer and mix a little bit in with your foundation," says Sonia. "Then use a synthetic brush to buff it onto the skin to give the face a beautiful tone."

highlighter: look radiant

Tip: One of my all time favorite products is an illuminator or highlighter. When you start to look ashy or gray, this little ditty will do wonders to make your skin radiant again. Who doesn't want that? That's why I love "strobing," the makeup technique of using illuminator to play up the best features of your face. It's basically the opposite of contouring. And boy, does it look youthful and pretty.

Try: Jouer Cosmetics Powder Highlighter, L'Oréal True Match Lumi Liquid Glow Illuminator, Anastasia Beverly Hills Glow Kit, and RMS Beauty Living Luminizer.

Technique: Illuminator or highlighter come in a mix of formulas and colors. I prefer creams because they blend beautifully, even on bare skin. Powders that have a shimmery finish can accentuate imperfections and make the skin look older. Opt for a shade that's similar to your skin tone: for pale skin stick with champagne or icy pink shades; for olive skin go with golden hues; and for dark skin choose copper or terra-cotta. Apply the highlighter only to the high points of the face, the places that naturally catch the light: along the top of the cheekbone up to the temples, below the brow bone, down the center of the nose, and above the cupids bow. Once the product is applied, blend in with your finger, fan brush, or a damp makeup sponge.

powder

Tip: Even if you're not a fan of powder, Ramy says that this is the time to make an exception and use it. Here's why: When you're sick, the last thing you have the energy for is putting on makeup. So, when you do, you're gonna want it to last until you get home and take it off. Dusting a little translucent powder over your BB cream or brow pencil—and your look will be locked into place. What's interesting about translucent powder is any makeup you layer on top of it also wears longer because the makeup adheres to the powder. "As a rule, I prefer pressed powder," says Ramy. "A loose powder gets in your eyes, all over your face. You have more control with a pressed powder. Plus you use less and it's still enough to set your concealer or foundation."

Try: Nars Light Reflecting Loose Setting Powder, Sonia Kashuk Undetectable Loose Powder, M.A.C Blot Pressed Powder, NYC New York Color Smooth Skin Pressed Face Powder, and Avon Ideal Flawless Pressed Powder.

Technique: When wearing translucent powder you need to be careful around flash photography. For some reason, the light reflects off the pigments. If you're heavy-handed with your powder, you stand the chance of looking like you have flour all over your face in pictures. You don't want to look like you belong in one of those horrible "Celebrity Makeup Fails" stories, do you? So, if you're going to a special event where flashbulbs will be popping, make sure to apply your powder sparingly with an extra large fluffy or kabuki brush. And never use translucent powder to catch errant eye makeup—it will look like you haven't blended in your concealer!

creating brows
and lashes from *scratch*

You know as well as I do, that the minute you lose your eyelashes and brows, shizz gets real. "I've had many women tell me that losing their hair—including their eyebrows and lashes—was more traumatic than losing a breast," says Ramy. "I've heard it a thousand times." The sad truth is that when you lose the hair on your face, you can't hide what's happening anymore. You lose part of your identity and your privacy, one eyelash at a time.

The good news—and yes, there is some—is this: "People have a lot of weird issues with their eyebrows under the best of circumstances," says Ramy. "And *everyone* has one brow that's better than the other." This plays to your advantage during treatment. "Most people are too busy worrying about their own eyebrows to be focused on what's happening with yours." The key is to do little things to improve the way your lashes and brows look. Don't drive yourself crazy, obsessing and trying to make them look exactly like they did before. That is mission impossible. Instead, a few easy tricks are all you need to make a big difference.

Tip: When you're experiencing hair loss, the best product to use is something made with crystalline wax like a brow pencil or pen because they adhere to the skin more than powder or liquid products. "You don't want your brows coming off at brunch," says Ramy. "With a wax-based product, you can be confident that when you put your brows on, they're going to stay on." A brush-on pomade (aka brow gel) is best for those who still have some hair because it is lightweight and helps fill in the sparse areas.

Equally important as the formula is the color of your brow product. If you still have some eyebrows, you want to choose a product that is a shade lighter than your hair. This will help fill in sparse areas while keeping the look subtle and natural. If your eyebrows are gone, opt for a color that matches, or is a shade darker, than what your hair color was or what your wig is. Ramy advises, "On bare skin you need a brow to be a bit darker for it to actually show up."

Try: Ramy Miracle Brow Compact, NudeStix Eyebrow Stylus Pencil & Gel, and Benefit Cosmetics Brow Zings Eyebrow Shaping Kit. "I love Brow Zings," says Joan Lunden, who used the kit when her arches went AWOL. "It comes with pigmented wax and powder and two tiny brushes. You dip the little angled brush into the wax to create the shape and then you use the other brush to apply the powder to set it in place. I like it because it really lasts."

Technique: When you don't have any hair at all, it might seem tricky to create brows from thin air. It will be intimidating at first. That's only natural. *The most important thing to do is to* let your bone structure lead the way. The structure of your brow bone predetermines the eyebrow shape that works for your face. If you have a square face, oval McDonald's-like arches won't jive with your

While there are basic beauty rules for looking your best, ultimately makeup should be something that makes you feel good. There is no question that this is a difficult time and doing your makeup will be more challenging than usual, but try to stay positive.

natural angles. Drawing anything freehand can be cause for the jitters, but these simple steps make it as easy as painting by numbers:

1 Hold your eyebrow pencil or makeup brush along the side of your nose. Where the tip of the pencil or brush meets your forehead is where your brow should begin. Use the pencil to mark the spot with a dot. Repeat on the other side.

2 To determine where the placement of the arch should be, Ramy advises, "Look where your brow bone protrudes the most. That's where the arch of your eyebrow should peak." Dot that spot with your brow pencil. Repeat on the other

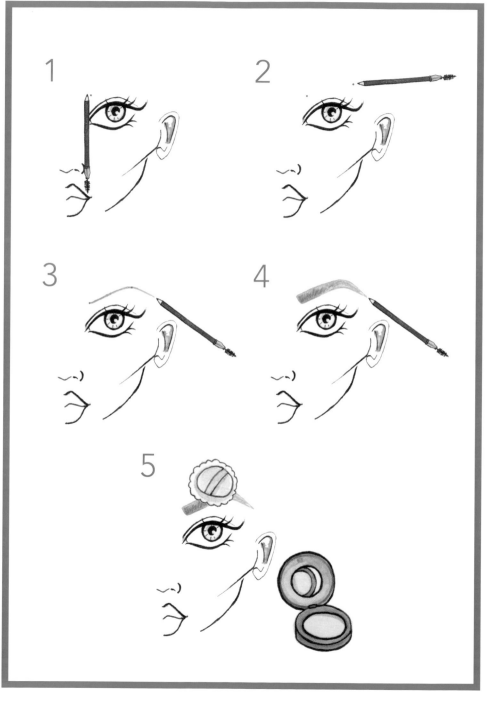

side. Another useful tip is to use a visual guide. Get a picture of yourself when you had eyebrows and use it as a visual reference. Tape it to the mirror and refer to it when drawing. It takes out some of the guesswork.

3 Begin drawing. Working from the beginning of the brow, connect the dots. If you are using a brow pencil make sure to sharpen it first so you get precise thin strokes. If using a makeup brush, opt for one that is thin with stiff, angled bristles. "Go to the peak in a straight line," says Ramy. "The line shouldn't curve or swerve at all. Just draw a straight line to the peak. From there, angle the pencil to the middle of your ear to draw the tail." If drawing your brows is too intimidating and you need a virtual cheat sheet, I swear by Ramy's Brow Master stencils. Unlike other stencils, these have adjustable inserts that allow you to customize the thickness, length, and width of your brows. All you do is adjust the shape, hold it against your brow bone, then fill in. It makes the job easy and goof-proof.

4 Once the basic shape is drawn, go back and begin to fill in the brow to make it look fuller and wider. Use little short strokes that mimic the look of individual hairs to make it as believable as possible.

5 If you are a little heavy-handed and the color goes on too dark or bold, take a little pressed translucent powder and pat it on the brows. This does a few things: it softens the color, nixes the waxy shine so your strokes of color resemble real hairs, and makes the brows wear longer.

tip: drastic times DO NOT call for drastic measures!

Don't go crazy trying to look the way you did before treatment began. Dealing with losing your eyebrows and lashes may be tough, but it's only temporary. Hair grows back. Don't do anything drastic, like tattooing your brows or lash line. (You'd be surprised how many women get permanent makeup during treatment.) Just give your body time, and things will get back to normal. Ya gotta give it a minute. Just chill.

lashes

Tip: When lashes are sparse or gone all together, rely on this illusion trick. "I apply eyeliner along the lash line, then smudge it out to diffuse the line," says Ramy. "This mimics the look of full lashes." While you still have some lashes to speak of, volumizing or thickening mascara is the best bet. It will help build up the width of the hairs so they appear more abundant.

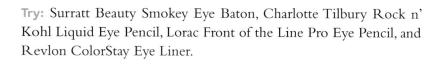

Try: Surratt Beauty Smokey Eye Baton, Charlotte Tilbury Rock n' Kohl Liquid Eye Pencil, Lorac Front of the Line Pro Eye Pencil, and Revlon ColorStay Eye Liner.

Technique: Opt for a creamy eyeliner that's easy to blend. Liner that is in the same color family as your hair will make the illusion of lashes more believable. Avoid using black liner as it looks harsh. Instead, earth-tone hues like brown, copper, and khaki are softer and more flattering.

Dot it along the lash line, then, very delicately, smudge it. Skip eyelash curlers, lash combs, and anything else that could pull on the hair.

fake it 'til ya make it

Tip: There is always extra pressure to look good when there's a big event to attend. Whether it's a friend's wedding, your birthday, or just a night out with the girls—a special occasion might require you to pull out all the beauty stops. What am I talking about—false lashes and eyebrow wigs! What are eyebrow wigs, you ask? They are individual human hairs that are grafted onto an ultra-light, skinlike fabric in the shape of an eyebrow. It's shocking how real they look. They come in four different eyebrow shapes—from a high arch to a straighter style, and in four different shades—from dirty blond to black. Eyebrow wigs are applied just like false eyelashes using a little adhesive glue. They can even be applied over existing eyebrows if your brows are just thin. The upside is that nobody will suspect they aren't yours because they flex with facial expressions and stay firmly in place even when swimming, showering, or working out.

Here's the caveat: The adhesive glue needed to apply false lashes and eyebrow wigs can be an irritant to skin during treatment. It's important to do a patch test to see if you will have a reaction to the glue or the remover before using them. Look for products that are hypoallergenic. If you don't have a reaction, then you're good to glam.

Try: Thrive Causemetics Kristy Faux Lashes (specifically designed to have a curve that hugs the eyelid so women without lashes can wear them), Ardell Demi Wispies False Eyelashes, Ardell Individual Flare Short Black, or Ardell 318 Lash Accents. Brow lashes can be purchased at HairPlaceNYC.com and Amazon.com.

Technique: Applying false eyebrows is pretty straightforward, especially if you keep in mind the placement techniques from earlier in this chapter. But I won't lie; applying false eyelashes can be a bit tricky, especially with fumbling fingers. The good news is that it gets easier each time you do it. Here's how:

Step 1: Choose a style that is believable. Opt for natural hair over synthetic. In my opinion, they just look more authentic and feel lighter. Also choose "natural" styles—ones that feature a row of individual, wispy hairs. My favorite brand is Ardell. Their lashes come in a variety of styles and can be purchased at any drugstore. But what I really love is that their website (www.ardelllashes.com) helps you choose the best lashes for your eye shape and color. It makes the selection process virtually goof-proof. Whatever you do, steer clear of the "glamour" lashes. These bold styles tend to be heavier and need to be adhered to natural lashes to stay propped up. They also just look over the top. The goal here is to fool those around you. Save the drag lashes for your post-cancer celebration.

Step 2: Pick the right glue hue. Believe it or not, eyelash glue comes in various colors. Brown and black glues are used to blend into the lid when creating a smoky eye. White glue turns clear when it dries. When you have few or no natural lashes, white glue is the best option because it is basically invisible.

Step 3: Liner before lashes. If you are going to wear eye shadow and liner, apply it before adhering the lashes. Applying makeup over a strip of lashes can cause them to come unglued, or worse, fall off.

Step 4: Have some tweezers handy. To apply your lashes, take a pair of tweezers and grab the strip firmly in the center. If the glue comes with a brush, sweep a light layer of it onto the back of the strip. If not, place a dab of glue on the back of your nondominant hand, then drag the base of the strip lightly over the glue. Wait about a minute until the glue becomes tacky to the touch, then apply to the rim of the lid.

Step 5: Perfect your application. Use the tweezers to apply the strip onto the edge of the lid. If you have lashes, they will help you guide the placement. Use the tweezers to adjust the placement, if needed. You have a few minutes before the glue sets, so don't panic if it's not positioned perfectly the first second you lay it down. To make sure they don't fall off, use your eyelash curler to squeeze the base of the lash strip against the lid. Don't squeeze too hard. Subtle pressure will do the trick to ensure the lashes adhere and are secured in place.

Step 6: Last, line the lid again. Reapply eyeliner, lightly, to help blend the base of the strip into your makeup.

hair growth *serums* and treatments

Many Cancer Cuties have reported great success in keeping their lashes and brows by using Latisse (available from Mylash in the UK) during treatment. Latisse is an FDA-approved prescription treatment for hypotrichosis (inadequate or lack of lashes). Originally, this topical solution was created to treat glaucoma patients. One of the side effects was that it made lashes grow like crazy. (If all side effects could offer up such beauty benefits!) After official studies were conducted, Latisse was officially approved as treatment for the lash-challenged. Latisse must be applied every night for sixteen weeks. My former assistant Monica tested this product for a story I was writing. She had stick-straight, sparse lashes. Within two weeks, her lashes were long and lush. The results were impressive, to say the least. And the bonus is that it can also be used on your brows. The only negative is that there are some serious side effects that come when using this product, including a possible permanent change in eye color and dry eyes. I suggest everybody, especially cancer patients, consult their doctors before using it.

If Latisse isn't your jam, there are a few other options—specifically Rogaine, Viviscal, and biotin—that can help get your brows and lashes growing again. Rogaine is topical minoxidil, an antihypertensive vasodilator medication that slows hair loss and promotes regrowth. Viviscal (a marine complex with minerals and vitamins) and biotin (vitamin B_7) are supplements that help strengthen hair and nails and encourage their production. For best results, they should be taken daily. But again, don't start any topical or internal treatments until you clear it with your oncologist.

pay attention to *expiration* dates!

Makeup is like the food in your fridge—every product has an expiration date. Of course, most of us don't pay attention to them. I don't know anybody who's gonna toss a Tom Ford lipstick just because it's over six months old. If they did, I'd think they were crazy. I, myself, am an admitted hoarder of lipsticks and eyeliners. I just can't seem to give them up. My Bobbi Brown gel liner will get cracked and dry before I'll even contemplate getting rid of it. With all the makeup on the market, it still seems like a total score when I find a lipstick, shadow, or mascara that works for me. Go figure.

Most products have an expiration date of three to six months. Some of them can be pushed to a year *if* (and it's a big *if*) they are kept clean. But—as I've said before—you're playing in a different ball game now. While in treatment, it's crucial to do everything you can to avoid an infection. Old cosmetics and dirty brushes may seem innocuous but they are often the leading cause behind cold sores, pinkeye, breakouts, impetigo (a gnarly group of pustules), and staph infections.

My general rule of thumb is to swap out my makeup at the start of each fashion season in April (spring/summer) and September (fall/winter). You wouldn't wear fall colors in spring and vice versa, so it just makes sense to clean and update your makeup at the same time as your wardrobe. If nothing else, it will help you stay on trend. If that seems too soon to part with some of your beloved beauty products, then try to follow the expiration guide below:

mascara: 3 months

Tip: The good news is that mascara has a built-in shelf life. When it's coming up on three months, most mascaras start to dry out and get flaky.

lip gloss: 6 months to 1 year

Tip: If you use a gloss with a silicone wand or bristles and wipe it clean after each use, you can extend use up to a year. Otherwise, update it with a new one after six months.

lipstick: 1 year

Tip: Here's a surprising fact: because lipstick is made with wax, it actually traps and harbors more bacteria than gloss. Cleaning it with a little alcohol after each use will help nix germs but it will also dry it out faster.

blush and foundation: creams, 6 months; powders, 1 year

Tip: Powder formulas contain zinc and titanium so they actually prevent bacteria from growing. When you see oil marks streaked across the top, if the color cracks or if it starts to smell—then it's time to toss. Foundations and concealers in airtight packaging, where you can pump or spray the amount you need, prevents bacteria from getting in the product and will help them last longer.

eye shadow: 4 to 6 months

Tip: Shadow is one of those items that if it gets tainted—or you think it could be tainted—you need to toss it STAT. No playing around with this one. Pinkeye during chemo, no thank you!

eyeliner and lip pencils: 1 year (or longer!)

Tip: Well, this is a bit of a shocker: products that you sharpen—i.e., pencils—can be used until the wee bottom. Why is that? Whenever you sharpen an eyeliner, lip liner, lip pencil, shadow pencil, or highlighter—you instantly remove any of the bacteria and dirt on the product. As long as you sharpen it after using, it will stay germ-free. Make sure to clean your sharpener after each use as well.

brushes and makeup bags: varies

Tip: Dirty brushes are often the culprits behind the bad things that happen to your skin. They act as a vehicle, transferring bacteria from your makeup to your face and vice versa. Similarly, your dark makeup bag can be a breeding ground for germs. To cut down the odds of an infection, I suggest three things:

1   Clean your brushes and tools weekly. When doing my laundry on Sundays, I also clean my brushes and nail tools. I wash them with Johnson's baby shampoo (a clarifying shampoo works just as well) and then I let them air dry on a towel. When brushes start to lose their bristles, it's a sign that the handle could be coming loose or corroding and it's time to replace it.

2 **Opt for a makeup bag that is washable.** I prefer the clear plastic designs because everything is visible, therefore easy to access. Once a week, when cleaning my brushes, I wipe down my cosmetic bag with warm soapy water. Cotton and nylon bags that are machine-washable are also good options. Avoid bags that can't be washed—like leather. Bags that are kept clean can be used until they fall apart.

3 **Use disposable sponges.** Like brushes and makeup bags, sponges can harbor bacteria. Even when a sponge appears clean, residue product and germs sit lurking within. And most are harder to clean than you might think. All the dermatologists, oncologist, and makeup artists that I interviewed for this book suggested using sponges that you can throw out after each use. It's cleaner and safer, which is something that's more important than having your contour on fleek.

tip: brush up on this!

Sonia Kashuk is known as the "Brush Queen" in the beauty industry. Beside her core collection of brushes, every year Sonia partners with an accomplished artist to create coveted, limited-edition makeup and tools that are truly objets d'art. "I've always been a big fan of brushes," says Sonia. "I feel like you can really get the most blended, polished look using a brush." Her go-to rule? "For cream products, stick with synthetic bristles. They don't absorb as much product and deliver a better glide. For powder products, natural hairs work best." To select the right size brush, use one where the bristles match the size of area where you will be working. "That gives you the most control."

color is *curative*

It might seem like looking pretty is an impossible feat when you've got mood skin and no eyebrows, but makeup can work magic. For most of us, the goal is to warm up your skin tone and give it some life. One of the most basic ways to do that is with color. "I started wearing royal-blue eyeliner," says Dr. Heidi Waldorf, dermatologist and breast cancer survivor. "I hadn't worn blue eyeliner in years, but when I started losing my lashes it just helped make my eyes pop." There's no question that it brightened her mood as well. "You want to use colors that make you look pretty and fresh," says Sonia. Her advice is to find colors that emulate your natural coloring. So, for example, if you want to find a lipstick that is flattering, look for a shade that mimics or is similar to the inside of your lip—rosy or berry-hued, rather than a classic red. To find the perfect shade of blush, pinch your cheek and the color that appears is the blush shade you should be using.

Often you will read or hear terms like, "blue-based" or "cool" colors versus "yellow-based" or "warm" colors. Blue-based shades are those whose formula is developed using blue pigments while yellow-based shades are created with yellow pigments. During chemotherapy, many cancer patients experience skin that turns sallow or green. If that happens to you, avoid warm shades including, orange, coral, peach, pale brown, gold, bronze, and copper. These will play up the yellow tinges in your skin and make you look sicker. Instead, opt for blue-based shades including pink, blue, berry, magenta, silver, and all the jewel-tones. They will help brighten your complexion and make you look healthy. That is the goal after all.

one final note: have *fun!*

While there are basic beauty rules for looking your best, ultimately makeup should be something that makes you feel good. There is

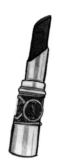

no question that this is a difficult time and doing your makeup will be more challenging than usual, but try to stay positive. If finding the perfect foundation is proving impossible or if dry skin is ruining your perfect application—don't get frustrated. Instead, find a way to make the experience something that puts a smile back on that pretty face of yours. Treat yourself to a private makeup lesson. Follow along with a YouTube makeup tutorial. Or wrangle some girlfriends to go lipstick shopping. When doing my makeup started to feel like a chore, I recruited some of my girlfriends to go explore the beauty shops in Koreatown, the neighborhood centered around West Thirty-Second Street and Sixth Avenue in New York City. There were so many cool cosmetics that I had never seen before that it got me excited to do my makeup again. Just remember: Keep it fun and simple. After all, being happy looks the most beautiful anyway.

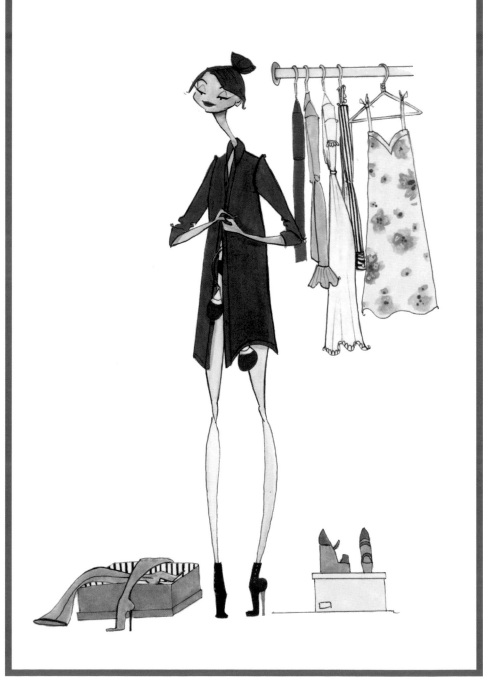

CHAPTER 8
THE BEAUTY OF STYLE

fashion that helps in the fight

At one point in my life—specifically when I was a fashion columnist covering runway shows and red carpets—I think I was pretty stylish. I loved reading *WWD* and the *New York Times* style section, shopping, and building outfits I would wear to work and out with friends. My closet was meticulously organized: shoes by heel height (flats, kitten heels, pumps, and then within their groups they were sorted by color). My clothes were hung by their categories: blouses, blazers, dresses, slacks, then suborganized by length and color (small black tanks on left, longer black shirts on right). Granted, this may seem next-level neurotic, but it made everything easy to locate and made me feel content. And even though I never had the budget to become a full-fledged fashionista, I always put effort into having a sense of style and looking put together. It brought me great happiness. That is, until I got cancer. Then everything changed.

I was lucky that during the first six months of cancer treatment I barely noticed any changes with my body. Other than the one-inch scar on my right breast and some slight bloating—you'd never know that I had had a lumpectomy or was in the midst of chemotherapy treatments. When I opted to get a mastectomy in lieu of radiation, I decided I was going to size up from an A to a C cup. Opting for bigger breasts was the chance for me to balance out my figure. Growing up I had a flat chest, "birthing hips," and a big ol' butt. While I wouldn't have gotten breast implants if I hadn't gotten cancer, they did help make my figure appear more proportioned. Thank you, cancer!

After surgery, I knew that my larger chest size would mean I would need some new tops and jackets. This, I expected. What I didn't expect was that Tamoxifen, the cancer medication I am required to take for ten years, would reshape my body completely. Three months after I started to take this drug I started to gain weight. While doctors report that the average weight gain is roughly three to seven pounds, I packed on almost fifteen! I am five foot one, so fifteen pounds turned me into the Michelin (Wo)Man. In hindsight, I didn't realize how much menopause would slow my metabolism and how sticky the weight would be. I kept eating and exercising in the same way I did before my diagnosis. By the time I realized how differently my body was functioning, I had become "curvy" (the nice way of saying I had exceeded my height-to-weight ratio).

With a wider ass, thicker thighs, and a muffin top in full effect, getting dressed became a whole new drama. Every time I opened up my closet, it was like a ghost of my former skinny, stylish self staring back at me. Every morning, like clockwork, I would have a major meltdown trying to squeeze into clothes that no longer fit. My tops were too small—no surprise there—but when I couldn't fit into my flowing skirts and baggy jeans, I would collapse on the floor in tears.

Body metamorphosis is tough regardless of the specifics. Some of you may lose weight and might not be able to pack it back on no matter how much pasta and how many pies you scarf down. Some of you may gain weight, then shed it after all the steroids and meds are out of your body. But for those of you who do experience a shift in your silhouette, I will be the first one to admit that it can be a frustrating hurdle. The good news is there are some very easy fixes. If you know to anticipate changes and head them off before they get out of control, then you'll be ahead of the game.

While other chapters in this book feature advice from the leading experts in their respective fields, this chapter I turned, mostly, to fashionable survivors to offer tips and tricks on how to dress your changing post-cancer body. They know better than anybody because they lived it. This is their advice, from the front lines…

dressing after surgery— recovering in *style*

After your diagnosis comes surgery. This, in itself, is overwhelming. And if you're anything like me, fashion is the last thing you are thinking about. But I am here to tell you that being prepared with some cozy clothes will make a world of difference.

After my mastectomy, I was sent home with two drains hanging from my breasts. (NOT HOT!) To say this was uncomfortable and clunky is an understatement. What made it worse was that I was woefully unprepared with clothes to wear over the drains. While in the hospital, the nurses advised me to get a few button- or zip-up shirts to make changing my drains easier at home. But when was I supposed to do this? After I was released and lugging around two plastic balls attached to my boobs? It would have been helpful to have this intel before I went in for my surgery. My neighbor Victoria came to my rescue, giving me a few old dress shirts, which were roomy and helped conceal the drains. The only problem was that they felt a bit stiff and were too baggy. Were they useful? Very. But in a time when I felt like I was slowly losing my femininity day by day, the shirts didn't help my emotional state.

Some of you may be sent home with drains. Some of you might have ports. Whatever your case may be based on the cancer you have—the one thing we all have in common is that we want to be comfy while recovering. An added bonus is looking even halfway decent. Here are some stylish tips for how to dress after surgery— whether in the hospital or at home:

lock down your loungewear

"The reality is, while you're recovering the place you will be interacting with people the most is at home on the couch," says Laura Rubin, diagnosed with stage II, HER2 positive breast cancer at age thirty-one. She is the founder and creative director of the communication agency, Left Left Right Consulting and creator of AllSwell notebooks. "I also had a boyfriend and didn't want to just let it all go. I took a look at my loungewear situation and it was really sketchy. So, before my surgery, I set a budget and went shopping for things I could wear that felt good against my skin but were kind of flattering. I didn't spend a lot of money but I purposely made it feel luxurious in a time when creature comforts are really important."

shopping list recommendations

Tank tops: If you have breast cancer, you won't be able to wear bras for a while so it's important to get "tank tops with shelf bras that have enough stretch and support," suggests Laura. Breast cancer survivor and Emmy-winning lifestyle expert Sandra Lee also stocked up on tank tops. "My reconstruction lasted almost a full year, so I had a tendency to cover up on top and wear things that weren't as revealing. Tank tops are really easy and they are also great if you are experiencing suffocating hot flashes." *tip:* Gap Body, American Apparel, and Victoria's Secret have a nice mix of affordable, flattering tank tops.

There is also a brand called Tender Tanks that was created by a breast cancer survivor named Carol Largent. The tanks have Velcro straps that make it easy to dress yourself without raising your arms and can be adjusted throughout the various stages of reconstruction. The tanks are also designed with wider armholes to accommodate drains and longer fabric in the waistlines so you can just pull the top down during doctor's visits without exposing your muffin top (www .tendertanks.com)!

Pajama sets: Opt for ones that button up in the front. And look for supersoft fabrics like cotton flannel. "It breathes and is really comfy," shares Laura. *tip:* If you're short on time, head to a department store such as John Lewis, which have large sleepwear departments stocked with a variety of options.

Robe: "I invested in a cute collection of bathrobes that I could just close over me while I was hooked up to my port," recalls Suleika Jaouad, diagnosed with aggressive myeloid leukemia at age twenty-two. She is a writer and *New York Times* Life Interrupted columnist. *tip:* Avoid hotel-style robes, as they tend to be bulky and will feel cumbersome when you are weak and tired. The best bet are those made with lighter moisture-wicking fabrics that dry fast and allow you to move freely and easily. The most scrumptious feeling robes are those made of terry cloth, silk, sweatshirt cotton, chenille, and fleece.

Slippers: Another unexpected necessity—slippers! "I had a big collection of slippers," says Suleika. *tip:* Stick with moccasin or booty styles that keep feet and ankles warm and offer the best support. Avoid mule styles as they tend to slip off easily and can be unsafe for those who are unsteady on their feet. I live for UGG's Alena slipper (it's also Oprah's favorite!). They are made with a soft suede exterior, plush wool interior, and a rubber outsole—so you can even wear them outside.

Blanket: "You want to feel luxurious tucked in your blanket while curled up on the couch," say Laura. "Mine was faux fur." *tip:* Blankies made of cashmere, cotton fleece, acrylic, and chenille are some of the softest ones out there. My favorite—hands down—is the Luxe Throw by Little Giraffe (www.littlegiraffe.com).

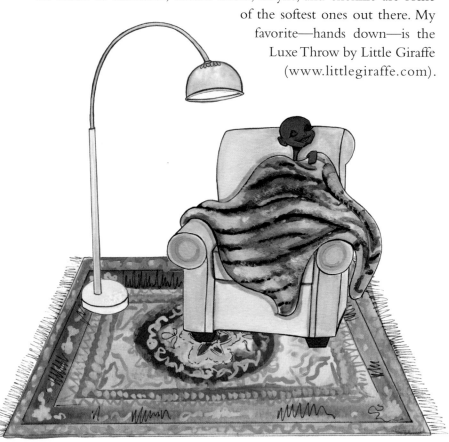

I got mine as a housewarming present and it's one of the most useful gifts I ever received. It certainly came in handy on the days after chemo when all I could do was lie around and watch TV. It's made from poly microfiber that feels *exactly* like chinchilla and is trimmed in satin. If you ever wondered what it feels like to sleep on a cloud, then wrap yourself up in one of these babies. It's heavenly.

tip: presents perfect for patients

"When you get sick people always want to know what they can get you," says Suleika Jaouad, myeloid leukemia survivor. "I always suggest cute pajamas that can be buttoned up or slippers. Someone gave me a cashmere hoodie that I never would have treated myself to but I wore it almost every single day for a year because the softness of the material on my bald head just felt so luxurious."

zip it up!

"Zip-ups are also very helpful while you're in the hospital. If you have any sort of port or tube that you have to be connected to at all times, taking sweaters on and off can be challenging. That's why I found zip-ups to be the perfect fix," suggests Dayna Christison, diagnosed at age twenty-three with stage IV nodular sclerosis Hodgkin's lymphoma. Now twenty-five, she has a thriving career as a model, creator, lymphoma activist, and cancer fighter. "Cardigans or button-ups work well too—as long as you feel comfortable in them. Zip-ups are a plus for us baldies while in hospital rooms because of the hood. I would always find that the air vent was inconveniently placed right above my head, which is the most sensitive to the cold."

don't be a boob—get the right bra!

For those of you who have breast cancer, finding the right bra is crucial. It helps hold your breasts or reconstruction in place so your incisions and stitches don't rip or tear. "I couldn't get my arms over my head after surgery to get a sports bra on. When I had my lymph nodes removed my arm was on fire. I was taking two or three painkillers at a time and it was still hurting—and I'm not a painkiller person," shares Torva Durkin, who was diagnosed with stage II invasive ductal carcinoma breast cancer at age forty-four. She is a wife, mother, and deli owner. "I found a sports bra that zipped up the front from Victoria's Secret—and it was amazing. What a difference that made. Front closure is key!"

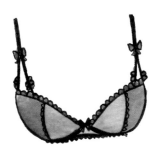

drain management

While a surgical bra is important, there is one thing I want to add to Torva's tip. If you have had a mastectomy—seven times out of ten your drains will be attached with safety pins. *Safety pins! WTF?!* I can't tell you how many times I pricked myself trying to reattach the drains after emptying them. Don't be a boob like me. Get the right bra before your surgery. One that I recommend is the Elizabeth Pink Surgical Bra by Best Friends For Life. This supersoft nylon-Lycra bra features a Velcro front closure, shoulder adjusters, and—*here's the important feature*—two side openings that your drains can be looped through. (See ya later, safety pins!) It is a genius bra that is easy to put on and take off to empty your drains.

There are other items that also help with drain management and might be better if you've had any of the flap reconstructions where you might have drains in other places on your body. If this is the case, there are fanny pack–like holders, robes, and hoodies that come with interior pockets specifically for drains. My recommendation is get one that fits your fashion needs during recovery. If you're hanging at home—a robe or bra will work fine. If you still need to put the kids on the bus or want to keep your bald head warm (like Dayna mentioned above), then the hoodie is the way to go. Below are some ideas and options:

* It's My Secret Post Surgical Jacket (www.itsmysecret.org)

* Marsupial Pouch (www.marsupialpouch.com)

* The Brobe Recovery Robe (www.thebrobe.com)

* Elizabeth Pink Surgical Bra by Best Friends For Life (www.bfflco.com)

don't be a style slacker

"I am a huge advocate of being comfortable while still looking good," says Dayna. "When full-set silk pajamas came into style a few years ago, I was all over it. When I was in the hospital, I had these fun, printed leggings in tie-dye and plaid that I would mix with an extra fuzzy sweater or an oversized graphic tee. I found that leggings were easiest for me because of the weight changes I encountered but I also had sweet leopard harem pants that I would wear around as well."

top recommendations

Fila: These leggings are a nylon-spandex blend, which offers the best of both worlds—stretch and breathability. They come in capri and full-leg styles so they can be worn in any season. Best part? When you are done wearing them in recovery, you can wear them to the gym (www.fila.com).

Plush: For the colder months, these leggings are the way to go. They are basic black cotton on the outside but lined with fleece on the inside.

And no, they aren't bulky. Even with the scrumptious lining, they remain thin and keep your silhouette slim (www.plush-apparel.com).

Buddha Pants: These are the softest, most comfortable and (surprisingly) flattering harem pants in the world. I didn't discover these until after treatment, but damn, I wish I had! The 100 percent cotton pant drapes beautifully, looks great wrinkly or ironed, and the elastic waist is a real savior (emotionally and physically) when your weight is fluctuating. But the best part is the patterns and silhouette of the pants will give you instant edge when you feel like you're experiencing a style low. Once you wear them you will realize what a gift this tip truly is (www.buddhapants.com).

dressing *during* treatment: baldies and changing bodies

During treatment, your dressing issues and fashion needs will be different than when you are recovering from surgery. Most likely, you are working or are interacting with people who require you to dress like it's business as usual. The most obvious issue during treatment is going bald. Wearing wigs every day can be a grind. But even if you don't lose your hair, dealing with a changing body can be just as overwhelming and challenging. How do you dress a body that looks and feels foreign to you? Here's how:

find ways to personalize your look

"When I first got sick, I was so lost. I was in a haze of doctors and treatment choices and the reality of my current situation that I felt so disconnected from who I was. It took me a while until I started to personalize my new look and what I felt comfortable in," says

Dayna. "It sounds silly but I would wear a beanie a lot because my head would get cold and to personalize it, I would scrunch it so that it was tilted to one side of my head mostly. It wasn't the most outrageous fashion trend that anyone had ever seen but I felt that it was something a little bit cool and different that I could play around with like I would my hair. Similar to head wraps! I personally felt really silly and out of my element when I would try head wraps but I feel like those would be a great way to mix it up and do a little something fun with creatively to add more 'you' to your look."

tip: color choice is key

When you lose your hair and are dealing with mood skin, color choice is more important than normal—especially when selecting face-framing accessories like hats, beanies, and scarves. "When you have no hair, pastels like baby blue and pale pink will make you look like a preemie. Literally, you will look like a baby. And black is too harsh when your skin is all weird," says Laura Rubin. "Instead, go for soft tones and neutrals, like gray, beige, and tan. They are most flattering for the face."

make accessories your essentials

By definition, accessories are secondary, smaller pieces that help complement and complete an outfit. But during treatment, accessories become major fashion players. When you don't have hair, when your waistline changes, or when your skin starts to look like a curiously colored opal, accessories function like magic tricks. Little illusions can distract from things you don't want people to focus on. Let's put it this way: Nobody is going to pay attention to your bald head if you're wearing a birdcage necklace with a live hummingbird inside. (Okay, this isn't realistic but you get the point...)

"I bought very expensive eyeglass frames. I had the optician add pads to the nose to lift it up so it would block where my eyebrows should be," shares Dr. Heidi Waldorf, NYC-based dermatologist and breast cancer survivor. "I also started wearing bigger earrings."

The message here: People are easily distracted. Give them something stylish to stare at and their attention will turn toward it.

Not the Noggin'! If you want people to stop staring at your bald head, opt for accessories that draw eyes away from your face. These include belts, shoes, bags, printed stockings, rings, bracelets, or a long necklace.

Miss That Muffin Top! If you want to distract from your fuller waist-line, swollen arms, or puffy legs, opt for accessories that draw eyes up to the face. Bold lipstick, bright eyeliner, big earrings, hats, and chokers work wonders.

treat yo'self!

I touched upon this piece of advice when talking about skin care ingredients a few chapters back but I think it deserves repeating now. Most of us live on budgets and don't have a lot left over once we are finished paying our bills. We pay our rent. We buy our kids clothes. We put food on the table. This is reality. However, there are moments in life when it's important to treat yourself. When your quality of life is just as important as your responsibilities in life. When I got sick, I splurged on really nice body and facial oils. It was a little treat that cheered me up in a big way. Every time I rubbed a drop of it on my skin, I felt less sick and less sad. This goes for treating yourself to some nice fashion items as well. "I started treatment during the winter and my head would get cold and my skin was really sensitive. You don't realize how much your hair keeps you warm. So I wore cashmere beanies by Alexander Wang. They were warm and made me feel better," says Laura. "In those moments, that's what matters, right?" I totally agree!

try to get dressed every day

"This is a hard one but it's important to try it," advised Dayna. "When I was recovering from my stem cell transplants, I felt my worst. I wouldn't get out of bed most days. I would feel crummy and I would look crummy. As a result, I would then get depressed about my situation. When I would get dressed to go to the doctors, though, I would feel better about myself—even when I was feeling awful. This may be challenging because of the physical state you are in, but if you can change into something other then what you went to bed in—like a comfy outfit that you can lie around in but still feel put together— you *will* see (and feel) a difference."

make your style intentional

"I am a pretty feminine gal and have always had long hair. So, when I was finally on the road to wellness but still had super-short hair, it was really difficult for me because I didn't identify with that girl at all," says Laura. "Still, I tried to play it up. I channeled my inner architect and played a little bit of a role. I wore cool wraparound glasses and created this alter ego, which was sort of fun. I made it look intentional. Even when I was wearing my beanies, I would choose ones with a little more volume to them, so that they hung off the back of the head like hair. Like I was one of those super-edgy girls with short hair and a beanie. The whole point was to make it look like an intentional fashion statement. I took control of the aesthetic and it made me feel less like a victim."

know this: pumps have power!

Cancer is a long haul. And the journey to wellness always lasts longer than anyone expects it to. The prolonged duration of time takes its toll on our energy, zapping our femininity, good looks, and style in the process. I mean, after three years of surgeries, treatment, and reconstruction, I barely had the energy to brush my teeth in the morning. But it's important to remind yourself of who you were—and still are. And never, ever, underestimate the power of a pair of pumps.

"As the days went along and turned into weeks, then months—I wasn't going out, I wasn't doing anything. One day, I looked at my husband and said, 'I think I can do this today. I think I can go out,'" says Elizabeth Myers, who was diagnosed with stage II invasive ductal breast cancer and BRCA2 positive at age forty-nine. So, she instructed her husband to get their van ready. "As I walked past my closet I saw what my girlfriend calls my 'fuck me heels' and I thought—'If you're going to do this, then really do it!' I grabbed a pair and sat down on my marble step in my foyer and put them on. When my husband opened the door, he grabbed his heart and said, 'Holy moly, look at my wife!' As a married woman, so much had been physically taken from me. But it wasn't just taken from me, it was also taken from my husband. He watched me go through the dregs of hell. The heels were important because I wanted to show him exactly how hard I was coming back, how ferocious I was, and what a sexy wife I could still be. He deserved it. I deserved it."

Heels are not comfortable but they do look SAH (sexy as hell). Even if you only have the energy to wear your four-inch stilettos while lying on the couch, none of your visitors will be looking at your bald head, chemo acne, or drain tubes. Instead, they will admire your courage, your spirit, and your sense of humor. More importantly, a pair of pumps will serve as a reminder that you are only a few steps away from being the gorgeous, glamorous woman you once were. Just keep putting one foot in front of the other and you will get there. This, I promise.

tip: a double-duty accessory perfect for "hot girls"

It used to be hard, if not impossible, to look chic when having a hot flash. That was until Connie Sherman created Hot Girl Pearls—a pearl necklace that helps you chill out when you feel overheated. The pearls are filled with a nontoxic cooling gel, which when frozen, can help stop your hot flash in, well, a flash. I am completely obsessed with these genius and gorgeous necklaces and bracelets. And they make a great gift for a survivor who is finding it tricky to stay sweat-free and stylish at the same time!

pull out a few hat tricks

Hair loss is one of the most devastating things to deal with during cancer treatment. As Suleika put it: "Hair informs our identity." Hair loss does too—and allows the world into our private lives, often against our desire or will. It really sucks. This is where having an assortment of head coverings comes into play, merging fashion and function. "At this point, I have more hats than anyone should own," says Joan Lunden. "They were a real lifesaver on so many levels."

There are some people who believe you need to follow certain rules to pull off wearing a hat. I am not one of them. Maybe your face shape would look better in one particular style but I think when you're up against cancer, you've got enough to contend with than to worry about some stupid fashion rules. Personally, I think you should wear whatever makes you happy—even if everyone else thinks it looks ugly as hell. That said, there are some head coverings that are better to wear during treatment. Below is the breakdown of the best options (and there are a lot!).

beanies

A small skullcap made from soft fabric that sits loosely on the head. Most cancer patients have one or two in their arsenal. Over the last few years, beanies have become popular with the fashion crowd, who wear them slouched back on the head. Look for ones with moisture-wicking fabrics like cashmere, modal, cotton blends, and soft furs including rabbit and chinchilla. Those with a fur pom-pom on the tip look whimsical and playful.

Steal: www.mychillouts.com. If you want a beanie that converts into a scarf try the Marmot Convertible Slouch Beanie, www.marmot.com.

Splurge: Fur beanies from www.adriennelandau.com

sleep caps

Body temperature drops during sleep so the head often gets cold at night. This is where sleep caps come in. These nighttime beanies have a supersoft interior fabric such as cotton, knit terry cloth, fleece, or poly blends that will wick away moisture and keep the head warm while you snooze.

The Go-to: www.headcovers.com

large-brimmed hats

These glamorous hats are often seen at the Kentucky Derby or on members of the British royal family. If you've never worn one before—now is your chance to get in on the action! While beanies and baseball caps are generally a top pick for those in treatment, a hat with a large brim is just as essential for blocking harmful UVA/UVB rays. When you are having chemotherapy, your skin is more susceptible to sun damage. These hats will shield your head, neck, and even the clavicle area from the sun, and make you look stylish at the same time. Talk about a win-win!

Steal: www.asos.com

Splurge: www.eugeniakim.com

trapper hats

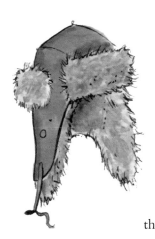

These Elmer Fudd–inspired hats aren't a typical go-to for cancer patients, but this is all I wore during the cold, winter months when I was in treatment. Here's why: They cover the entire head including the nape of the neck and have flaps that also cover the ears for serious insulation! While the outside can be a mix of fabrics, typically wool plaids or brushed suede, the interior fabrics are plush fleece, softened sheep's wool, or alpaca hair. Bonus: with the flaps down, it hides the fact that you don't have hair!

Steal: www.furhatworld.com

Splurge: R&V is the brand that I wear—leather on the outside, fur on the inside. All-around deliciousness (www.rv-hats.com).

cloche

The great thing about this vintage-style hat is that the bell shape provides optimum coverage for the face and neck. It sits low on the head, covering the forehead, and fans out slightly by the ears. For those who have a retro vibe, this is hat that will complement your style.

Steal: www.hatcountry.com

Splurge: www.ericjavits.com or borsalino.com

fedoras

This classic hat looks amazing on just about everybody and is guaranteed to turn heads whether you're wearing it casual or dressy. But more than any other hat, it's important to try on a fedora before buying for two reasons: 1) They are typically made with stiff wool or straw, so it's important to make sure the fabric and feel won't irritate your scalp; 2) Without hair, your head will be smaller—so you probably won't wear the same hat size that you did before. Trying on the hat will ensure it fits properly. If you already have a fedora you want to wear, but now feels roomy, tie a silk scarf on your head and knot it in the back, then wear the fedora over it. JLo does this all the time and it looks super stylish.

Steal: Lack of Color (www.polyvore.com or www.nordstrom.com)

Splurge: Rag & Bone (www.rag-bone.com)

turbans

This head covering is constructed with long sheets of fabric that wrap around the head and gather together in front at the top of the forehead. While this is a very specific look, it is a great way to mix up your style. Elizabeth Taylor rocked them frequently in her day. Today, fashion icons including Kate Moss, Karolina Kurkova, Beyoncé, Eva Mendes, and stylist June Ambrose wear them. "I collaborated with this turban line called Robin Hoods. They are easy to tie, easy to wear and didn't make me look like a psychic or tarot card reader," says Suleika. "Plus, they are less cumbersome than a big hat."

Steal: www.robinhood.com or www.topsyturban.com

Splurge: www.shopstyle.com

baseball and newsboy caps

Baseball caps are casual, fun, and easy. Those with an adjustable strap in the back are great for wearing over wigs. Others have built-in extensions that give the illusion that you have a head full of hair when you don't. "On the inside is Velcro all the way around the hat and you get one with hair attached or you can put in your own extensions," says Joan. "And then you take the fake hair and pull it into a ponytail so it just looks like you put on a baseball cap and your hair is pulled back. Nobody knows a thing. And it's not terribly expensive. I found these really helpful." But be warned: Even though baseball and newsboy caps have large front brims, they leave the neck, ears, and bottom of the face exposed to damaging UVA/UVB rays—something you will be more sensitive to during treatment. I suggest you wear them indoors only. If you want to wear them outside, make sure you slather on your sunblock!

The Go-to: www.hatsandhair.com or www.hatsforyou.net

berets

This classic French hat is much like a beanie, except that it is round in shape and hugs the head. It is intended to sit on the top of your head or off to the side. The downside about a beret is most are constructed in wool-based fabrics that are great at wicking moisture but tend to be extremely itchy, hot, and constrictive. That said, if you have a beret you love (like I do), here's how to make it less itchy: Buy a large square piece of soft-moisture wicking fabric and sew it in as an interior lining. (If you use small snaps or thin Velcro, instead of sewing it in, you can remove the lining to wash it.) Choose a dark color so that sweat stains don't ruin the look.

Steal: www.asos.com or www.simons.ca.com

Splurge: www.netaporter.com or www.saks.com

head scarves and bandanas

I always suggest that my fellow cancer patients carry a scarf around when in treatment because they are so multifunctional they can help out when you least expect. Among the uses: they keep the neck warm during chemo; they can conceal a chest in transition; and the most obvious—they hide a bald head! Survivor Torva Durkin shared her cold cap headscarf tip back in Chapter 2—make sure to check it out (on page 60)! Most scarves are made with silk, which will slip on a bald head. I suggest fabrics that have a little texture like modal, bamboo, or cotton blends.

Bandanas—the smaller cousin to the head scarf—offers similar functions with a more casual vibe. "I found these bandanas online that aren't an actual triangle and are specifically for bald people," says Joan. "It looks like a regular bandana but with an elastic back so that if you are outside and the wind blows, that little flap doesn't fly up and expose your bald head. That can be kinda embarrassing." To make your life even easier? Opt for a scarf or bandana that is pre-tied.

The Go-to: www.curediva.com

dressing your post-cancer bod

To me, this is a big issue that nobody ever talks about. Everyone had tips and suggestions for me during treatment but once I was in the clear, it was radio silence. I didn't have a clue on how to begin dressing my new body. Every day that I woke up and looked in my closet, it induced pains of anxiety and depression. You can avoid that with the following tips:

do some spring cleaning (whether it's fall, winter, or summer...)

There is nothing worse than opening up your closet only to stare at clothes that don't fit you. Besides taking up space, they get in the way of picking out your outfit in an efficient manner. For me, it was also emotional clutter. I would pull out a dress and a flood of memories would flash before me—images of when I was healthy, skinny, and pretty. Talk about a bum-rush.

"I lost a pretty drastic amount of weight. I went from being a fairly curvy, busty young woman to one that was rail thin. None of my clothes fit anymore, so the most important thing for me was to take all the things that no longer fit me and get them out of my closet. They just made me feel worse about the way I looked and what was happening to my body," shares Suleika. "I did a big spring cleaning and put all the clothes in a duffel bag, which I put in storage. I tried to turn it into an opportunity to do some fun shopping with my girlfriends and my mom. But it's important to really minimize what's in your closet to the things that make you look and feel good."

I know it can be hard to let go of items you love. It took me over a year to finally make the move myself. After all my clothes were folded neatly in garbage bags, I sat on my bed and cried. But once I dropped them off at the Goodwill, I have to admit, I felt freer. "You have to use the principle of feng shui," says stylist Daniele Hollywood, who has worked as a costume and wardrobe designer on *The Good Wife* (seven seasons), *Law & Order* (thirteen seasons), and now the new

CBS show *BrainDead*. "If it doesn't serve you and it's causing you emotional blockage, you have to let it go. Give it to someone else who needs it. That opens the door for something new to come into your life."

plan your outfits

This sounds so basic, but planning out your wardrobe in advance, when you aren't watching the clock, will help nix those frenzied moments in front of the closet trying on skirt, after skirt, after skirt. After a million morning meltdowns, one Sunday I stopped this negative cycle by creating a week's worth of outfits. I continued to do this, until I was used to and comfortable dressing my new body.

Another part of planning your outfits is shopping for them. If you've ever been bathing suit shopping, you know it doesn't always end well. I am not a great shopper. Department stores overwhelm me—there's just too much selection. I do much better after a "drunk brunch" with my closest girlfriends. We sip a few bloodies, eat eggs Benedict, and then hit up Zara. This takes the edge off and allows me to have fun. Part of taking care of yourself after cancer is avoiding *anything* that can leave you feeling frustrated or depressed. Figure out what shopping style is most enjoyable for you. You'll be happier and more fashionable as a result.

find your uniform

The good news is fashion rules are passé. Now you can wear white after Labor Day. You can mix prints and patterns. You can even rock those pretty silk pj's you've been wearing around the hospital to a cocktail party (not that you would want to). This gives you carte blanche and street cred at the same time. And now is the time to take full advantage of this fashion freedom.

"Because my body was changing so drastically, I no longer

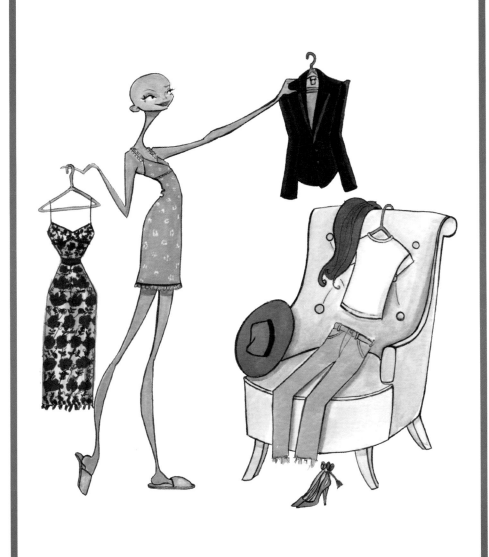

recognized myself in the mirror. The flowing dresses and heels and things that I wore before my illness no longer fit with the person staring back at me," says Suleika, now twenty-eight. "I wanted to feel tougher and a little bit braver and this gave me the opportunity to experiment with new styles. So I started adopting an edgier uniform. I bought a leather jacket. I bought boots with spikes on the heels. I think what I was looking for was some sort of armor—and I found it through fashion."

Don't have a clue on how to find your uniform? Let your figure guide you. "One of the tricks of the trade is to find a silhouette uniform," says Daniele. "Find something that flatters your body type and that feels good on you. Then stick to that. I do this even for all the actresses I dress."

When in doubt, leggings and flowing tunic tops always work. The top provides enough room to move comfortably while concealing any physical changes or surgical apparatus including ports, drains, even colostomy bags. The leggings help slim your figure.

But that isn't the only trick.

"This has been and always will be the most important tip to me as a breast cancer survivor who had both breasts removed and no reconstruction," says Elizabeth. "What can you do about not looking flat-chested if you choose not to wear padding or prostheses breasts? My trick is wearing blouses, shirts, and tank tops that have ruching, overlays, or are adorned with designs that have a 3-D effect. They add volume where there isn't some naturally while being fitted along the waistline so you still have a bit of a figure. Long, chunky necklaces and scarves also create the illusion of a bust. It's all smoke and mirrors."

how to wear (not eat) chicken cutlets!

If you are like Elizabeth and opt out of reconstruction, breast prostheses will help you regain your former shape and symmetry. There are two main types of prostheses:

Silicone: Looks and feels the most realistic. Most women opt to wear silicone prostheses to work or while having sex because it is the best at mimicking the weight and movement of a natural breast. There are three silicone subtypes:

* **Asymmetrical:** Designed only for the right or left side.

* **Symmetrical or pear-shaped:** Designed to work on either side and can be worn centered to create the cleavage and fullness or sideways to round out the outer portion of your bra.

* **Custom-made:** These are for women who have special needs—like large breasts or a skin tone that can't be matched with the existing offerings. A plaster cast or laser scan is taken of your chest and then silicone or latex prosthesis is made.

Foam or polyfill: These lightweight prostheses are best when you want a form that isn't heavy or hot. "I would wear these when it was hot outside or when I wanted to exercise," says Elizabeth, adding, "Sometimes, I would just take shoulder pads from old clothing I had from the eighties and attached them inside a strapless dress. Silicone prostheses are heavier and if you have a dress without straps, you can't keep it up."

Foam forms can be worn in salt water or chlorine—but be advised—they tend to want to float. "We have a big pool in my back-yard and one time my then twenty-five-year-old son hoisted me across the pool and my prosthesis came floating up before I did," recalls Elizabeth, who can laugh about it now. "My advice is make sure to buy a swimsuit with a prosthesis pocket built in." These pockets can also be found in lingerie, camisoles, and tops. Other options include adhesive patches or magnets that hold breast forms in place. The adhesive patches attach at the top of the form and can be worn without a bra. The downside to this is that the adhesive has to be replaced every week. Forms that have a magnet on the back sit it place with the help of an adhesive magnet that attaches to your skin.

If you're like me and believe "the devil is in the details," there are also faux nipple forms that can give your breasts a very realistic (i.e., perky) look. Pink Perfect, a company founded by breast cancer survivor Michelle Kolath-Arbel, makes realistic, ready-made and custom adhesive silicone nipples for women who have undergone unilateral or bilateral mastectomies. Each style comes in various skin-toned hues including soft pink, coral, peach, sand, tan, brown, chocolate, and mahogany. They are also waterproof and can be worn in the shower, ocean, or swimming pool (no floaters, hallelujah!). The faux nips come with a nontoxic sensitive glue that keeps them adhered to the skin for up to four weeks before they need to be reapplied. The ready-made styles range around £200.

Get the right fit: If you opt to go the prosthesis route, a breast care nurse will arrange a fitting appointment for you, typically at a local NHS hospital. While you can buy breast forms at a host of stores, Elizabeth suggests going to specialty bra or lingerie boutiques where they have trained professionals to help you get the proper fit, color, and shape. She also suggests bringing a few pieces from your wardrobe—like a blouse, dress, or swimsuit—to make sure the form looks good in all your clothes. "Let's say you had on a very gauzy silk blouse, if you lean or move in that blouse with normal breasts, you see the fullness, the roundness, the weight of that breast. So you need that weight in a prosthesis to work inside your clothes properly."

Get reimbursed: NHS patients do not have to pay for their prostheses. If you are private and do have to pay, ask the fitter to sign a VAT exemption form stating that you have had breast surgery.

look cool—even with hot flashes

If your treatment put you into menopause, dealing with hot flashes and night sweats will be an issue. While there isn't much the doctors can do to change this situation, there are a few fashion tips you can use to minimize how miserable it can be.

Fabric choice is key: Cotton is a popular fabric because it's soft and it's easy to care for. That's why it's a bit surprising that it's *not* the best option when dealing with hot flashes. While 100 percent cotton "breathes" beautifully, it is also hydrophilic, which means it absorbs water. While it is amazing at sucking moisture away from the body, it also retains that water so your clothes look wet longer. Instead, opt for cotton blends and moisture-wicking fabrics including jersey and cotton-jersey. Another great option is modal, the fabric used to create most yoga clothing. It is made from reconstituted cellulose from the beech tree and considered part of the rayon family. It is supersoft, smooth, breathes well, and dries fast.

Dress in layers: This is an obvious one, yet many of us do it wrong. Here's how to get it right: *The first layer,* the one closest to your body, should be made with a moisture-wicking fabric. I find that a nice camisole or tank top with shelf bra is best because they look polished and are work-appropriate, even if you need or want to remove your other layers. *The second layer* should be 1) loose enough to allow the air to flow around your body; 2) lightweight so that in case it gets wet, it will dry quickly; and 3) easy to take off. *The third layer* is about keeping warm when you aren't having a hot flash. Lightweight fabrics that trap heat, like cashmere and silk blends, will keep you comfortable temperature-wise without adding or creating extra heat around your body.

Prints and patterns? No sweat! Illusion tricks are super helpful when dressing during and after cancer. This is one of them: If you are suffering from hot flashes, prints and patterns in bright colors are a great way to hide perspiration stains. Avoid solid shades, especially light neutrals like gray or tan, which show every drop of moisture.

tip: sheets for night(mare) sweats

Night sweats are just as bad as—if not worse than—hot flashes. They soak your pajamas and your sheets and disrupt your sleep in the process. I can't tell you how many nights I woke up at two a.m. soaking wet and had to change my pj's, then strip and remake the bed. It's the worst. Make sure you have a waterproof mattress cover to keep your bed dry and clean. I also advise getting sheets made of moisture-wicking fabrics. Wild Bleu makes bedding with Heat Release Technology that pulls the moisture away from your body and allows it to evaporate (wildbleu .com). They cost £££ but they'll save you ZZZs.

Don't drink the Hatorade!: Most of us are guilty of being too harsh on ourselves about our physical appearance. As a society, we have unrealistic expectations of what we should look like and the clothes we should wear. It puts a lot of pressure on us. And it's a real burden for cancer survivors. So, I'm here to tell you that it is really important to put a cap on the negative internal dialogue about your changing body. Your waistline may not be the same. Your body might resemble a road map thanks to the scars. Even your hair will be different. But you f★cking survived!!!!

"You can't let the negative talk pull you down the rabbit hole," says stylist Daniele Hollywood. "The fact is, nobody has a perfect body. Focus on what you like about your body, enhance that, and then just be kind to yourself." I agree!!! You spent all this time and energy beating cancer and now you're going to start beating yourself up? Do you know how crazy that is?! At the end of the day, confidence and a smile are the only things you really need to wear to look your best anyway! Put them on and be proud of yourself!

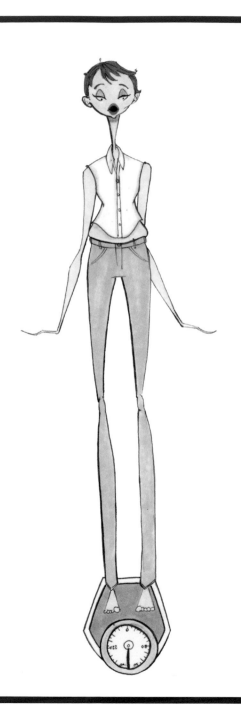

CHAPTER 9

LIFE AFTER TREATMENT

Congratulations, beautiful!!!!! You made it to the other side. Now that all that nonsense is done, it's time to celebrate! If you are anything like me, you haven't spent a lot of time thinking about what happens now. I get it—you've been a little busy having surgery, heading to chemo and radiation appointments, and basically living in your doctor's office. The good news is you are now, officially, a survivor (holla!!!). That alone, makes you friggin' fabulous!!!

Getting used to your post-cancer body requires a bit of an adjustment period. For me, this was the toughest part—partially because I felt unprepared for how my body changed from chemopause (chemically included menopause). I'm not going to lie, some of the physical changes really suck. I want to spare you the drama; being prepared is half the battle. Whether it's dealing with hot flashes or weight gain—all are manageable. Listen, you handled cancer like a boss—this is nothing compared to that. You got this, girl!

bye-bye estrogen, *hello* menopause!

It was about six months after I started taking Tamoxifen that I started to see a difference in my physical appearance. I had made it up until that point pretty much resembling my old self—except, of course, for my new knockers. I felt pretty good too—all things considered. But once I was in full-blown menopause, my hair texture changed, my nails began peeling and breaking, my skin lost its resilience and glow, and hot flashes would leave me dripping in sweat—several times a day. And if that wasn't bad enough, my girly bits became as dry and lifeless as the Sahara. Talk about adding insult to injury!

I don't say this to scare you. But menopause is often a shitty side effect caused by chemotherapy and cancer drugs, including Tamoxifen or aromatase inhibitors. While my doctors told me to anticipate menopausal changes, I wasn't really prepared for how they would play out. By the time it was in full effect, I felt like I was living in a remake of *Revenge of the Body Snatchers*. I didn't recognize my body anymore.

I came to learn, over time, that this is a common feeling among survivors. At first, I thought the struggles were singularly mine. But once I started talking openly about it and writing articles on hush-hush topics—I *instantly* learned that I wasn't alone. In fact, I learned that I was luckier than most. Many of our sisters experience really harsh side effects—some even painful. Surprisingly, there are some easy things you can do to mellow the harsh.

But first, let's take a step back: What's actually happening in your body?

"Menopause is when you have a loss of estrogen and all the things that estrogen helps," says Dr. Heidi Waldorf, dermatologist and breast cancer survivor. "Estrogen helps reduce wrinkles. Estrogen helps improve elasticity and keeps the collagen healthy. It keeps your skin hydrated and plump. It keeps your hair growing in the right places and not the wrong places. It also helps maintain that very sensitive vaginal mucosa."

Everyone's menopause experience will be different. How your body reacts depends on a few variables including your age and the overall condition of your health at the time of your diagnosis. Regardless, many survivors worry about the long-term physical effects of treatment and cancer drugs. It's a valid concern. When faced with skin that seemed less resilient, hair that appeared dull, a slower metabolism, and a dry vagina, I was alarmed. And that's putting it mildly.

cancer drugs *101*

By now, you've probably heard about Tamoxifen or the class of drugs called aromatase inhibitors. But what are they? How do they work? What are the side effects you can expect when you start on them? To help answer these questions, I turned to Dr. Jennifer Litton, a breast medical oncologist at the University of Texas MD Anderson Cancer Center—one of the top nationally ranked cancer institutes in the United States—to give us the 411.

Let's start with Tamoxifen. Tamoxifen is a pill generally given to premenopausal women. It can also be used by postmenopausal women, but only when aromatase inhibitors don't work or cause side effects that impede quality of life issues. "Tamoxifen is a selective estrogen receptor modulator," says Dr. Litton. What does that mean? "Basically, it is very similar to estrogen. It binds to a lot of those receptors that estrogen would normally bind to and feed those tumor cells. But it binds there, it doesn't feed the tumor cells, and it doesn't get out of the receptor. It just sits there. So the cells starve off because they are not getting the estrogen."

Women who are already in menopause when they are diagnosed or for those who are induced into menopause either with shots or because they've had their ovaries removed, are put on an aromatase inhibitor. There are three: Arimidex (generic name: anastrozole), Femara (generic name: letrozole), and Aromasin (generic name: exemestane). "Aromatase inhibitors shut down the final formation of estrogen that you make outside of your ovaries," says Dr. Litton. "So, for postmenopausal women, even though it's low, I think that's a big surprise that women still make estrogen in other parts of their body—like in the fat cells. Aromatase inhibitors have a completely different mechanism of action than Tamoxifen. What they do is shut down the last chemical conversion. Tamoxifen sits and binds to a receptor and sits there like the flag that sees the estrogen."

While the functions of these drugs are very different, the side effects are largely the same. They include hot flashes, weight gain, vaginal atrophy, joint aches and pains, and a decrease in bone density. "One of the things not really in the literature but that I've seen with these drugs is some hair thinning too," says Dr. Litton. "Sometimes that can be really upsetting."

Whether you experience any—or all—of these side effects depends on so many variables. The good news is that each can be managed. Let's talk about the ones that can mess with your beauty mojo.

feelin' the *heat*:
hot flashes and night sweats

There is still debate in the medical community about what causes hot flashes and night sweats. The Mayo Clinic points out that not all women who lose estrogen also experience hot flashes or a shift in body temperature. What the evidence does show is that menopause-driven estrogen loss is linked to changes in the hypothalamus. The hypothalamus is an almond-sized area in the brain that regulates body temperature, hunger, thirst, fatigue, and sleep—among other things. The leading theory is that when there is a decrease in estrogen in the body, the hypothalamus detects it as too much body heat. The brain's natural response is to release hormones that lower the body temp, which causes the heart rate to rise and blood vessels to dilate to allow more blood to flow through and dissipate the heat. The increased blood flow sets off the body's natural cooling method: sweat. This series of events—the heated, flushed sweaty situation—is what we call a "hot flash" or "night sweats," depending on the time of day they happen. Bottom line: a.m. or p.m.—they are uncomfortable, irritating, and inconvenient.

While hot flashes and night sweats are out of a woman's control, there are some things that bring them on or make them worse. To help minimize your hot flashes, it's important to pay attention to the things that could be triggers. To help lessen the number and severity of hot flashes, try avoiding:

* Alcohol

* Caffeine

* Spicy foods

* Sugar

* Stress

* Smoking

* Wearing tight or heavy clothing

One surprising thing I found that helped my hot flashes was a bit of unexpected intel I learned from Dr. Larry Norton, medical oncologist and the deputy physician-in-chief for breast cancer programs at Memorial Sloan Kettering. Dr. Norton was giving a talk at the 92nd Street Y in Manhattan when he said some women found that their hot flashes were more manageable when they switched the *time* that they took their Tamoxifen. He said that when these women took their pills at night, rather than in the morning, they reported shorter, less severe hot flashes and night sweats. He was quick to add that there was no scientific data to back up this claim but for women struggling with this side effect, it might be worth trying. I was one such woman and started taking my pill that very night. Within two weeks my hot flashes, and especially my night sweats, started to subside. While they didn't go away entirely, they aren't as hard-core as they were before.

Dr. Litton also adds a little tidbit of encouraging information, "For most people, hot flashes are most pronounced the first five or six months and then often they get slightly better," she says. "I really try to encourage my patients to get through those first months because it gets easier after that."

weighty matters:
taking a pounding after cancer

I never had a muffin top until I started taking Tamoxifen. A year into taking the anticancer drug, I walked past my bedroom mirror only to catch a glimpse of my belly jiggling. I almost had a heart attack. No matter how hard I worked out—three or four times a week—I couldn't shed the weight. Studies show that the average weight gain from hormonal changes brought on by Tamoxifen or an aromatase inhibitor ranges from "seven to ten pounds," says Dr. Litton. Because estrogen levels are lower, it makes fat harder to shed. This "sticky weight" generally settles around the abdomen. But cancer drugs aren't the only culprit. The natural aging process plays a role as well, slowing the metabolism and diminishing muscle mass and bone density, among other things. When your body is forced into menopause all of these things happen at the same time—and the effects can be startling.

Here's the thing you don't want to hear: It is imperative that you are disciplined with your diet and exercise. Before cancer, it used to be a cinch for me to shed five pounds in less than two weeks if I was strict with my food and workouts. Today, my muffin top hangs around like an ex-boyfriend I can't seem to ditch. Anything that disappears into my mouth, shows up on my waist within days. It's a cruel existence.

Here's how to manage it like a pro.

make a nutritionist part of your squad

When you are being treated for cancer, you will have a team of medical experts overseeing each phase of your care. A nutritionist should be one of them. Most patients either don't think to consult with a nutritionist or don't want to deal with going to one more appointment. But a nutritionist's advice and guidance can make a huge impact on how you look and feel during and after treatment. Most, if not all, cancer hospitals have nutritionists on staff who are there to help you create meal plans and shopping lists, and provide recipes when your taste buds and food restrictions will be at their worst. They are also there to help you figure out how to adjust your diet for life after. My advice is to make the most out of your trips to the hospital by piggy-backing your appointments. After you see the oncologist, stop by the nutritionist's office. You can also make use of the hours you are sitting in the chemo suite by having the nutritionist come to you. Either way, the sooner you can get on a healthy eating plan and establish good habits, the better it will be for your look—waistline, skin, nails.

minute on the lips = lifetime on the hips

You've heard this expression a hundred times but it's especially true after cancer treatment. After I was diagnosed, I decided I was going to make myself happy by eating all of my favorite foods. "Cheat nights" became everyday "treat nights." Chicken scarparelli, enchiladas suizas, and pizza (duh) became regular meals in the Kiernan household. And pretty soon, they became regulars on my stomach, thighs, and arms. I think dealing with cancer is two-fold: You have to be kind to yourself and give yourself a break. On the other hand, you have to remember that you are going to live, so you can't throw in the towel like there is no tomorrow. You have to maintain a sense of control so you can main-tain a sense of yourself in the long run. Consider this: Once you are on drugs that will put you into menopause, you will have to eat about two hundred calories less per day just to maintain your pre-cancer weight. And that doesn't even take into account the additional weight you will gain from treatment. The less you consume, the less weight you will gain. It's that simple. Treat yourself, but do so in moderation. I still allow myself "treat nights" with meals that have a higher calorie counts than Bill Gate's net worth, but I limit them to weekends or a night out. Trust me when I say, making a disciplined choice of salad over pasta is *waaaaay* less painful than the hours you will have to log in at the gym to burn off the calories later on.

shake what your mama gave you!

Working up a sweat is going to keep your bod healthy and hot. But hitting the gym or heading out into the great outdoors for a brisk walk has more benefits than just losing or maintaining your weight. More than a hundred epidemiologic studies prove that thirty to sixty minutes of moderate to vigorous exercise per day drives down the risk of reoccurrence. The findings also show a 20 to 30 percent risk reduction, which is even higher for postmenopausal women. Here's why working out is such an effective anticancer tool:

★ Estrogen doesn't just come from your ovaries. It is also produced and stored in fat tissue. The more excess fat you have, the higher the level of estrogen that remains in your body. This leads to the development of more fat tissue and more estrogen. It's a vicious cycle that ups the chances of your cancer coming back.

★ Exercises triggers apoptosis, programmed cell death, helping kill off cancerous cells *before* they become cancerous.

★ Physical activity increases circulation of the blood and lymph systems. If you've ever heard of, or had, a lymphatic massage, then you know how important it is to "get your juices flowing." While the circulatory system relies on the heart to pump blood through our bodies, the lymphatic system (made up of tissues and organs) relies on exercise to flush out the body's toxins and waste, called lymph. Lymph nodes help "catch" or filter cancer cells that might be floating in the fluid in the body. This is why surgical oncologists remove some of the nodes located in the armpit during breast cancer surgery. Examining them helps doctors figure out the extent of the cancer in the body. When we sit on our asses and don't move around, those toxic, acidic liquids pool around the tissue and can cause issues like lymphedema.

* The loss of bone density is an expected side effect of menopause. Weight-bearing exercises help build muscle and bone mass and strength, reducing the risk of osteoporotic fractures.

* Exercise can limit the intensity and length of hot flashes and night sweats.

* Working out boosts your brain's feel-good neurotransmitters, called endorphins, which reduce stress and elevate your mood. Working up a sweat in the gym will ensure you "don't sweat the small stuff" in the rest of your life.

the effects of cancer on your (whispered voice here)...*vagina!*

It amazes me how nobody prepares you for how your vagina is going to change once you have cancer. Most of us are so focused on the battle and the area of our body that is being gutted by the cancer that we don't even *think* to ask about our vajajays. Well, prepare yourself, because cancer treatment and menopause brought on by chemo or cancer drugs change things—drastically. Normally, the vagina is lubricated with a thin layer of clear fluid. The physical evidence of this is what we call "discharge" often seen in the lining of our underwear. Estrogen helps maintain that fluid and keeps the walls and lining of the vagina healthy, thick, and elastic. When estrogen levels bottom out, the fluid dries up and the lining and tissue become thinner and less elastic. This is called vagina atrophy, vulvovaginal atrophy, and genital

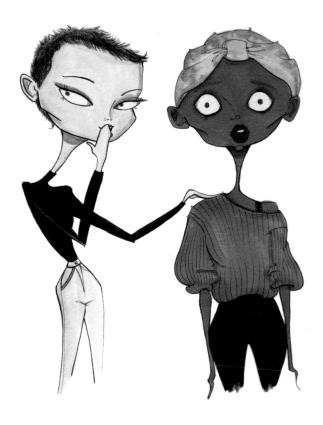

urinary syndrome menopause.

This can be the toughest part of being a survivor. The hits just keep on coming. As an editor, what saddens me the most is that many doctors and the media really don't want to talk about this life-altering side effect. Survivors are often left to grapple with the issue alone. I can't tell you how many times I have pitched this topic to my editors only to have the line go dead the minute they hear the word "vagina." What the f★ck is this, 1950?

In a day and age when a celebrity sex tape can launch a *Vogue*-cover career, why is it still taboo to discuss a dry vagina after cancer? It's our responsibility as survivors to force this dialogue and remove the stigma once and for all! We have a right to the information—especially when it impacts our quality of life.

My vagina got dry after chemo. Soon after, I couldn't achieve an orgasm without a lot of work. I felt "dead" down there. As a single woman, it was a nightmare. I am not alone.

According to published studies, 90 percent of cancer survivors

> **According to published studies, 90 percent of cancer survivors will experience some form of vaginal atrophy and sexual dysfunction. 90 percent!!!! That's almost all of us!**

will experience some form of vaginal atrophy and sexual dysfunction. Ninety percent!!!! That's almost all of us!

And you know that if this were a male-related issue, there would be a pill for it by now.

"Let's talk about survivorship because the chances are your doctor never ever talked to you about your sex life beyond cancer," says Dr. Lauren F. Streicher, associate clinical professor of obstetrics and gynecology at the Feinberg School of Medicine at Northwestern University and the medical director of Northwestern Medicine Center for Sexual Medicine. She is also the author of *Sex Rx: Hormones, Health, and Your Best Sex Ever* and *The Essential Guide to Hysterectomy*. According to Dr. Streicher, the most common side effects include: decreased libido, affected arousal, limited orgasmic ability and dyspareunia (painful intercourse), bleeding—oh, and this doozey—chemotherapy-induced oral mucositis in the genital tract. "The mucosal lining in the mouth is similar to that of the vagina so it makes sense that patients could get sores there," she says. "But nobody ever tells you to expect that or what you might do to treat them when they occur."

That's true of most of the topics centered around this part of your body. Here's information that can help.

the sahara syndrome: dealing with a vagina as dry as a desert

Since a dry vagina is at the root of a lot of these problems —including itching, bleeding, and painful intercourse—let's start here. The most obvious fix is lubricants. "All lubricants are not created equal," says Dr. Streicher. "I steer women away from water-based lubricants particularly if they have propylene glycol in them because they tend to get sticky and gloppy and irritating. The post-cancer vagina does not need anything that is going to be irritating." She recommends Pre-Seed (a lube for couples who are trying to conceive) because it is the least irritating for cancer patients with inflamed tissue. Unlike most lubricants, Pre-Seed does not harm sperm and helps mimic cervical fluids—so its great for couples who are trying to conceive after cancer. However, it is contraindicated for women like myself who have estrogen-based cancers. But not to worry! There is another great option: Replens Silky Smooth, a vaginal moisturizer often mistaken for a lubricant. "You put it in the vagina twice a week and it makes the water absorption in the vaginal tissue increase," she says. "In many women it works as well as a local vaginal estrogen. In the clinical trials, the biopsies of the vaginal tissue showed the same changes/results."

corpse crotch—damaged, diminished, and feeling "dead" down there

It's not just survivors in chemopause that will experience changes to their vaginal tissue. Women who have had pelvic radiation to treat cervical, vulvar, rectal, anal, or uterine cancers will also experience changes in the shape and size of their vagina and the vaginal tissue.

Lubrication won't fix this. What will? "Right now, you have a number of different options," Dr. Streicher says. "One is using a local vaginal estrogen product." These come in many forms—creams, gels, lubricants, and now even serums. Among the most popular picks: Vagifem (a pill inserted into the vagina), Estring (inserted vaginal ring), Estrace (cream), Esphina, and the soon-to-be-released Lasovoxigen (serums).

Now, I know many of you who had estrogen-based cancers will think it's too risky to use an estrogen-based product. I felt the same way. But Dr. Streicher says the science proves these products are safe to use. In her book *Sex Rx: Hormones, Health and Your Best Sex Ever*, Dr. Streicher cites a paper published in *Breast Journal* that calculated the total amount of estrogen delivered in one year of using a local vaginal estrogen product. I would like to share her intel because it is important that the FACTS of this issue—not the fear—lead the conversation:

> *Vagifem delivered 1.14 milligrams, with an average blood level of 4.6 picograms per millimeter. Estring delivered 2.74 milligrams, with an average blood level of 8.0 picograms per milliliter, and Estrace cream had a maximum yearly average of 7.1 milligrams, with a variable blood level (since doses vary). As a point of reference, the average serum estrogen level in a postmenopausal woman who takes no estrogen is 10.0 picograms per milliliter or less. Women who take systemic estrogen therapy take one milligram each day. Women who use a vaginal estrogen take one to 7 milligrams per year.*

During our interview, Dr. Streicher added this interesting tidbit: "I did a survey of 1,000 academic female gynecologists and I asked them, 'If you personally had an estrogen-positive breast cancer and had problems with vaginal atrophy would you personally use a local vaginal estrogen for the rest of your life?'" she says. "Ninety-three percent said yes, they would." As with all medical issues like this, be sure to check with your doctor before using any sort of local vaginal estrogen to make sure they're right for you, but these findings are certainly encouraging.

For those who opt out of using estrogen-based products, there are a few other things that can help.

use it or lose it

The first one is a DIY. "There is something to be said about 'use it or lose it,'" says Dr. Streicher. "We know women who are having intercourse on a regular basis tend to have better lubrication and elasticity than women who've had a long hiatus." Most of us battling cancer go months—if not the entire duration of treatment—without having sex. That's normal, so don't knock yourself. But don't be surprised when you get frisky again that you have a Sahara Situation down below. "One thing women can do proactively to keep the tissue elastic is use a Rabbit-style vibrator," she advises. "The Rabbit is a penis-shaped dildo with an external component for clitoral stimulation" that helps you get revved on the inside and out. Talk about a win-win.

laser focused

The second thing that can help are lasers. "Lasers in my vagina?" you ask. As crazy as it sounds, that's exactly what I'm talking about. Most of us are aware of the use of lasers in cosmetic dermatology. Instead of having to go under the knife for even the smallest nip and tuck, lasers allow us to lift, tone, tighten with little (and in some cases, no) downtime. Hence, their popularity and expensive price. But these lasers aren't just for the face. Now, doctors are also using them to reinvigorate the vagina. Whether you've had a baby, are getting older, or are in post-chemo menopause, these lasers are nothing short of miracle workers. They tighten the vaginal tissue, minimize incontinence, restore moisture, and heighten sensitivity. Within the last few years, four new noninvasive lasers have launched in the United States: MonaLisa Touch and FemiLift (fractional $CO2$—just like Fraxel for the face), IntimaLase (YAG lasers), and ThermiVa (radio frequency).

Fractional CO_2 lasers use a beam to create microscopic cuts in the vaginal lining. As the wounds heal, "the physical response is an increase in blood vessel growth and collagen in the supportive tissue," says Dr. Elizabeth Eden, a New York City–based gynecologist in private practice and president of the New York Gynecological Society. Dr. Eden is also the clinical assistant professor of gynecology at NYU School of Medicine. "The end result is thicker, stronger vaginal walls, an increase in moisture, and an improvement in atrophy and laxity." A side benefit is that the pH levels and natural bacteria even out—so women experience less urinary tract and yeast infections.

Radio frequencies lasers, like ThermiVa, use controlled heat to warm the tissue until it contracts and tightens. While the fractional and YAG lasers can only be used on the inside of the vagina, lasers using RF can also be used on the outside to tighten the labia majora. This is a big benefit for those who want to tighten up everywhere after childbirth. While research is ongoing to determine which of the lasers deliver the best result, early reviews recommend MonaLisa and FemiLift for atrophy and ThermiVa for tightening.

The procedure for each laser is slightly different but each starts like a regular gynecological visit—with the patient reclined and their feet up in the stirrups. The doctor inserts a wand in the vaginal canal and sweeps it 360 degrees with pulses of energy. Each laser session varies between five and twenty minutes. To get the best results, three sessions, spaced a month apart, are required. One "touchup" session is recommended once a year or on an as-needed basis. Some of the lasers also have a one-time fee for the wand that will be used during each appointment. Unfortunately, none of these are covered on the NHS.

(Quick side note here: I understand these laser treatments are a big out-of-pocket expense and not in everyone's budget. I wish there was a cheaper alternative. One of the reasons I wrote this book was to help share information about the latest treatments and products that have quality-of-life benefits. These lasers do. My opinion is that they should be covered by insurance for cancer patients because they aren't "cosmetic" procedures but are used to improve a survivor's physical (and emotional) health. I encourage you to write a letter urging your congressman or senator to push for insurance coverage for these treatments. It's our responsibility as survivors to make the journey easier for those after us! (Stepping off my soapbox now...))

So...the big question: Does it hurt? I had the FemiLift laser treatments and I can tell you from personal experience—there is absolutely no pain whatsoever. How can that be? "The nerves that innervate the vagina are not the kind of nerves that send a signal to the brain that says it hurt," says Dr. Eden. "They are not traditional pain receptor nerves that you have elsewhere on your body."

The only downside—for me—was that I couldn't have sex for a week after each treatment. Which, let's be honest, is not really that big of a deal. I could still work out, bathe, and proceed with life as normal. And I saw and felt immediate results. It has made a huge improvement in the health of my vagina and my sex life. And while I still keep lube on the nightstand, it isn't the slip 'n' slide situation I required before. The laser treatment has allowed me to get back in touch with a part of myself that had been missing since my first chemo session—a part of me I thought I'd never feel again. And I couldn't be happier about that.

Cab to VSPOT Medi-Spa: $23

Three FemiLift Laser treatments: $2,500

Reusable laser wand: $200

Moist, youthful vagina: Priceless

getting your *booty mojo* back

There is nothing like cancer that puts a serious damper on your sex life. I'll admit, it's hard to feel sexy and "in the mood" after having had your tits taken off and toxic chemicals pulsed through your veins. I wanted no part of it. Plus, I was just flat-out tired. When I was done with reconstruction, I thought I might get back on the horse (so to speak), but just as things were winding up, along came menopause. Before I knew it, I had no libido and was having trouble achieving an orgasm. This was difficult to deal with. A lot of the survivors I talked with shared similar experiences. And it's even harder when intercourse is painful. Local vaginal estrogens will help bring your vagina to the party, but you may still be hesitant to join in the festivities. "Menopause does affect the ability to become aroused," says Dr. Streicher. "Lower levels of estrogen decrease blood flow to the vagina and the clitoris—and that can be a roadblock to achieving orgasm." So, what will help? Here are some of her suggestions:

keep your eyes on the prize

If you are having a hard time achieving the "big O," don't let it get to you. Often, when we focus on what's not happening, it actually prevents it from happening. You hear stories about women that really want to get pregnant but can't. Then, the minute they adopt a baby, they get pregnant. It's the same thing. Don't be your own cock-block. It might take work but it will happen.

don't keep secrets

Your partner isn't a mind reader. If you don't let them in on the secret that you are having a difficult time getting in the mood or achieving an orgasm, they won't know to help, let alone be able to. Sharing this news can be scary but it will encourage the both of you to be more patient—maybe even more playful—in bed. This advice also goes for your doctor. They can help—but only when they have the intel.

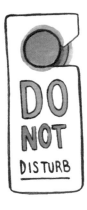

werk it

Dr. Streicher said it best before: "Use it or lose it." There is scientific evidence that women who masturbate on a regular basis have an easier time achieving orgasm. Since blood flow to the vagina and clitoris lowers after treatment and menopause, self-stimulating will help keep the blood flowing there. Doing it when you are alone will make it easier when you are with your partner.

try pelvic floor therapy

If painful intercourse and/or incontinence are issues that aren't being resolved with local vaginal estrogens or lasers, try pelvic floor therapy. This specialized physical therapy targets the muscles, ligaments, connective tissue, and nerves that support the bladder, uterus, vagina, and rectum so they can function properly. "Orgasms require contraction and release of the pelvic floor muscles," says Dr. Streicher. "So, if achieving an orgasm is an issue, these exercises can help with that. They can also help make them stronger and last longer."

As a survivor, every day is a new experience, especially when getting used to my new body. But even with all the changes—most of which are admittedly unpleasant—I feel stronger—both physically and mentally—than I ever did before. You and I have powered through what will probably be the most difficult thing we will ever face in our lives—and we are still here living life, laughing, and looking good. I'd call that a win.

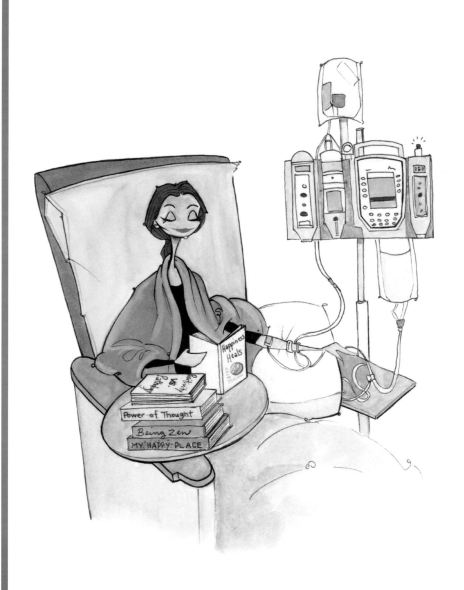

CHAPTER 10

HAPPINESS IS A STATE OF MIND— RELOCATE THERE!

We've all heard that having a positive attitude can have a positive effect on your health. Just some of the articles and books I've read claim that an upbeat attitude can help increase healthy cell proliferation, boost the autoimmune system, and halt tumor growth. If only this were true…

The problem with being positive is that it can be a double-edged sword. A patient who believes that a positive attitude has the power over their prognosis might feel pressure to be in a good mood and keep a smile on their face at all times. This isn't realistic when dealing with cancer. What happens if that patient tries to be positive and their treatment doesn't go according to plan? They might blame themselves. "In 2010, there was multiple meta analysis of a lot of these studies and most didn't find a causative relationship between positive thinking and survival," says Dr. Mindy Greenstein, psycho-oncologist, clinical psychologist, and consultant to the psychiatry department at Memorial Sloan Kettering. Dr. Greenstein is also a breast cancer survivor. "For a while, people were really pushing specific kinds of attitudes on cancer patients and it was just another pressure for them."

Sadness, guilt, fear, anger, depression, anxiety, hopelessness— these are all *very* normal emotional reactions when battling cancer. Trying to ignore them will make you feel worse—emotionally and physically. Forcing a positive attitude can actually backfire by creating stress that takes an added toll on the body. Dr. Greenstein says that her mentor, Dr. Jimmie Holland, calls this, "the tyranny of positive thinking."

So—let's keep it real. Forget being positive! There are better ways to handle your feelings. We will get to them in a minute…but first, a story.

As most of you know by this point in the book, a year before I was diagnosed with cancer, I had major spinal fusion surgery. During my four-month recovery, I was home on disability and basically had to relearn how to walk. It was the worst time of my life. Until that point, I was a pretty negative person. From the time I was a child, I was sassy and argumentative. By the time I was in my twenties, I was cynical and jaded and always saw the glass as half-empty. This attitude did not work in my favor when I was recovering from back surgery. The natural fear and worry anybody would experience after a major health crisis coupled with a fatalistic attitude sank me into a deep depression that brought me close to committing suicide. Quite honestly, the only thing that prevented me from killing myself was that I was pessimistic about succeeding. Oh, the irony.

So why am I telling you all this? When I was diagnosed with cancer, I vowed that I would approach this health crisis with a different attitude. I knew I had to flip the script if I was going to survive—not just physically, but emotionally. To do that, I decided I was going to retrain my brain. Every time a negative thought crossed my mind, I would shut it down and find the silver lining in the situation. Losing my hair? I get to wear wigs that let me try new hairstyles without commitment! Gaining weight? Now I have an excuse to wear my comfy sweats 24/7! When a bad thought entered my mind, I found a happier or funnier one to chase it away. At first, this required a minute-by-minute presence of mind. And boy, was this work! When I *really* started paying attention to each of my thoughts, I was shocked by how negative I was. But as I put this practice into action, day by day it became less of an effort and more automatic. My mind would catch itself and switch the thought.

But here's the thing: I wasn't trying to replace negative thoughts with positive ones. For me, the trick was to find something beneficial— like a life lesson or a gained perspective. I didn't force myself to be happy. Many days, I wasn't. Many days, I mourned for my old life, my old body. But even in those moments, I had a greater awareness, and hence an appreciation, for my life. The life I was still living.

"What's important is that we all have a trial-and-error system of figuring out what works for us," says Dr. Greenstein, author of *The House on Crash Corner*. "Rather than focusing on having a positive attitude, which can be very, very murky, focus on the things that make you feel better. That's what you need to do more of."

Translation: Find your happy. Whatever makes you happy— indulge in it and indulge often.

"Everyone knows when your brain is happy; it gives off good stuff like endorphins," says Hoda Kotb. "Feeling good, feeling happy—and not pretending that you feel good or just saying you're happy—but really being happy helps your brain give you more of that good stuff that helps you along the way. So much of it is mental. When you feel better and happy on the inside, the rest of it kind of works."

> *My point being, is that going rogue, hopping the rails, switching gears—whatever you want to call it—can actually set you on the right path. The path that was intended for you.*

Dr. Greenstein recalls a story about one of her patients who had a terminal diagnosis. He was hoping to live another five or ten years but refused to stop drinking and smoking. "I said to him one day, 'You know, you're still smoking and drinking,' and he looked at me and said, 'Listen, I'm dying. You want to take away my candy?'" recalls Dr. Greenstein. "You know what, he had a point. It wasn't a good thing but he was looking to enjoy whatever time he had left. He did not get his five years but he lived on his terms and enjoyed the time he had, which I think is being positive also."

So, are we condoning you go out and start boozing and whooping it up? No. Don't be daft. What we are saying is that life is about living. And you aren't living life unless you are enjoying it. So, I do advocate going rogue a little if need be. I did—and not just by a little.

Here's how that went down:

By the time I was in the middle of chemo, I had had a lot of time to contemplate the direction my life was headed. I was unchallenged at work. I was sad and resentful being in a relationship with a man that wouldn't commit. I didn't volunteer and had no hobbies to keep me interesting or make me a compassionate person. I wasn't living the life I wanted to live. I wasn't becoming the woman I knew I could be. During my reconstruction, one persistent thought sat in the corner of my mind: *This is your second chance in life to get it right—make changes now!* This thought nagged at me for months. Then, one day as my supervisor started irrationally screaming at me (something she did regularly), I had had enough. After nine years of reliable, loyal, dedicated employment—I quit my job on the spot. A week later, I broke up with my boyfriend. And a week after that, I started writing this book…

My point being, is that going rogue, hopping the rails, switching gears—whatever you want to call it—can actually set you on the right path. The path that was intended for you.

Today, I am a TV beauty producer and am blessed to work with talented people who teach me every day and who value my talents. I found the love of my life, my soul mate. And I pursue my passion projects—you are reading one of them now. Thank you for that!

So, how do you find your happy while battling cancer? As a cancer survivor and psycho-oncologist, Dr. Greenstein knows first-hand. These are her insider tips.

figure out your *coping* style

"Some of us have a more realism-based way of coping. We need to know all the facts. We need to know what to expect and then we can deal. Some of us have a denial-based way of coping, which is to just say 'Everything's going to be fine,' whether that's true or not," says Dr. Greenstein. "None is superior over the others." So, why does it matter? Knowing what coping method complements your personality can help you handle crises with a greater sense of ease and will give you peace of mind as a result. The main coping styles include:

* **Task-oriented coping:** This technique focuses on targeting the source of the stress and eliminating it or learning how to manage the stress associated with it. Those that cope this way seek advice on how to deal with their stress, have a plan, take action, focus on the positives, and are realistic about the situation.

* **Emotion-oriented coping:** This technique is when a person relies on external strategies—like yoga, meditation, or going to church/temple/mosque to pray—to manage stress. Research shows that emotion-oriented copers have less doubt in their minds and experience less anxiety.

* **Avoidance-oriented coping:** This technique is when a person copes by displacing emotion on others, wishful thinking, drug use, gambling abuse, risky behavior, or ignoring the problem. It is also called maladaptive coping. (*tip:* Even though Dr. Greenstein says one coping style isn't better than the others, my advice is *don't* use this one.)

get a *mantra,* then get *chanting!*

According to research done at Cleveland University, rhythmic tones involved in chanting create a melodious effect in the body called neurolinguistic effect (NLE). When we chant a mantra that has special meaning to us, it creates a psycholinguistic effect (PLE) on the body. The NLE and PLE effects are by-products of the production and spreading of curative chemicals in the brain. The research concludes that this is the reason why chanting provokes curative effects in the mind and body. Here's how it works:

Each tone vibrates the bones, muscles, and fluids of the chanter. The elongations of vowel sounds are particularly healing to the brain and the body. But even if it's a phrase you are repeating, it will take on a melodic rhythm that works the same way and offers the same benefits.

Brain waves begin to balance after three or four minutes and the temperature of the muscles and skin rises. (Warmer temps keep the muscles and skin pliable, soft, and in a state that is more conducive to healing.)

Research shows that when the body is in a state of stress, anxiety, depression, or anger, the natural variation in cardiac rhythm becomes weak and erratic. The research also shows that when we repeat mantras, or prayers, we automatically adjust our breath to six or fewer breaths per minute. What's important (and cool) to note is that this is the *exact* frequency and natural rhythm of key biological functions including heart rate, blood pressure, and blood flow to the brain. This synchronization of biological rhythms and functions has serious benefits including promoting a healthier immune system, reducing inflammation, regulating blood sugar levels, and lowering blood pressure.

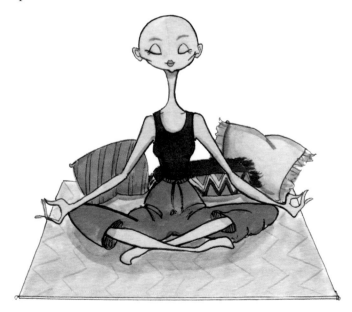

remember to *breathe*

"Some things are very, very simple and sound silly but remembering to breathe—just slowing down—helps," says Dr. Greenstein. "One thing that people have found helpful for a range of issues, including cancer, is mindfulness meditation or mindfulness-based stress reduction (MBSR). There are apps specifically for guided meditations. I use Headspace because I love the voice of the guy who leads the meditations." Much like chanting, studies prove there are many physical and emotional benefits to meditating. However, the most important benefit is that it helps quiet the mind when your hard drive is in overdrive. A quiet mind is a peaceful mind.

call on your girl gang

"One of the most helpful and necessary factors for coping well in a crisis is having a social support system," says Dr. Greenstein. "Who makes you feel better? Who helps you feel gratitude and appreciative? Who reminds you of what's meaningful in your life? Surround yourself with those people."

I can't agree more with Dr. Greenstein on this point. I don't know what I would have done without my Girl Gang when I was sick, with both my back problems and cancer. There was a period of three very dark years, and they were the only things that kept me distracted and sane during that dreadful time. Each one of my friends, in their own unique way, saved me. On days when I couldn't get up, my sister Moira would hoist me out of bed, into the shower, and dress me. On days when I couldn't see straight through the stream of tears, Carly and Dana got me to laugh, hysterically. When I went freelance and didn't have steady income and was stressed to the gills, Leah assigned me story after story, some that included traveling to some pretty dope locations. When I didn't have the energy for anything but sitting on

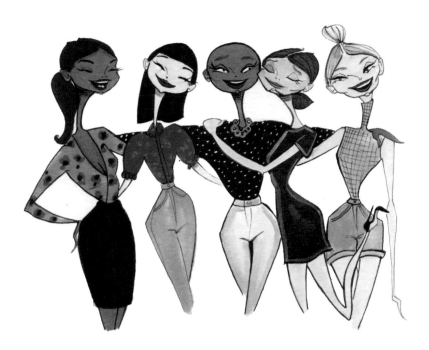

my couch, Jesse would drive three hours to watch hours of bad TV and carb load on salty chips with me. When I needed to get away, Nicole flew me to California and propped me up by her mom's pool while my other gal pal Juliette had me over for slumber parties with her baby boys. These women were my guardian angels on earth. I emerge from this battle a warrior only because I had the most loyal, devoted soldiers by my side. I owe them my life and I love them to death.

I recommend you lean on your girl gang as much as I did. Be aware that your friends might not be sure how to help or what to do. Most people get nervous or scared that they will say or do the wrong thing—so they end up doing nothing. It's not that they don't *want* to help. They don't know *how*. I encourage you to be vocal. Need a meal delivered or want some company? Tell them! I promise that before you hang up the phone, your doorbell will start ringing.

"E" is for exercise!

I mentioned the importance of exercise in the last chapter but what you might not know is HOW important it is for you, especially now that you have cancer. Extensive research proves that thirty to sixty minutes of medium- to high-intensity exercise done three to five days a week can cut the risk of getting cancer and halt it from reoccurring. A joint study released by Harvard Medical School and Women's Hospital in 2012 showed that one in ten cancer patients die from lack of physical activity and it is responsible for more than 5.3 million cancer-related deaths globally. The study, which was first published in *The Lancet*, goes on to state that "physical *inactivity* has become a contributor to the burden of disease and shortening of life expectancy comparable to smoking tobacco." What???!!!! That is crazy.

Personally, I hate working out. It's the last thing I want to do with the five free minutes of personal time that I have. So, I try to make it a fun social activity. I rope my friends and colleagues into attending aerial yoga or spin classes with me. I get my boyfriend, Kenny, and his kids to go on hikes or scenic walks. Anything to mix it up. I still hate it but I do it. Beside the obvious benefits of a smaller waistline, increased energy, and a lower risk of depression/anxiety/stress, exercise also has a dramatic impact on healing your body after surgery—making it heal eight times faster! I don't know what else you need to hear. So, get your tuckus up, slip on your cutest gym outfit, and *get moving!!!*

give yourself a *break!*

Most of us live by deadlines, obligations, and goals. Setting high expectations can be a good thing when it drives us to excel, but in most cases a checklist of objectives just adds unnecessary pressure and stress. It's a lot to manage. When dealing with cancer, it's important to wipe the slate clean of anything you don't *need* to be doing. Making your life as simple as possible—for the time being—will allow you to focus on getting healthy. "One of the most important things to do—and it's amazing how hard this is for many people—is give yourself a break," says Dr. Greenstein. "Cut yourself some slack."

When I was diagnosed, my job as a beauty director required me to do a lot of business dinners with beauty brands, PR people, and experts. It was my job to discuss how we could partner together to promote their projects and increase the magazine's revenue streams. These dinners would extend my workday and keep me out very late. When I got sick, I felt the need to continue doing all aspects of my job to keep up the status quo. My bosses didn't make me feel this way. It was my own self-imposed pressure to keep things "normal."

But as my chemo treatments revved up, I had to face the fact that things weren't normal. I didn't have the energy I once did and I needed to preserve what was left to help my body heal. After a lot of internal dialogue, I blocked out my calendar so nothing could be scheduled after work hours. I was anxious about this at first, but by prioritizing my health, the things that really mattered in my life quickly came into perspective. Sometimes, you need to step back, step away, to see the full picture. "I often hear patients say, 'I'm not doing it right. I should be more active. I should be more this or more that. I should be better,'" says Dr. Greenstein. "There is no right way to cope or deal with cancer. Adding that pressure is only putting hurt on top of hurt. You gotta let it go. Do what feels right for you. Do what makes you feel better."

This doesn't mean you should drop all your responsibilities like they were hot potatoes. If it's your day to pick up the kids—then pick up the kids! And if you are the type of person who needs a healthy distraction to stay sane and you still have the energy, then, by all means, keep busy! But it's important to recognize when things aren't working for you and to give yourself permission to say "no" to them. If doing the food shopping is one chore too many, recruit a friend to help out. I began ordering from Fresh Direct so that I had one less chore to do each week. If your volunteer gig is draining you of energy, tell them you're taking a temporary hiatus and you'll see them again in a few months. Unless it is an obligation that means life or death—and there are very few of these—then it can be rescheduled, reassigned, or removed from your checklist. When something makes you feel burdened, stressed, or overwhelmed, then it's time to say "no." And when you do—it's important to not beat yourself up about it. Be selfish—this is the one time it will serve you well.

while you're alive—*live!*

Dr. Greenstein touched upon this tip with the story of her patient who kept smoking and drinking until he passed away but I'd like to expand on this thought a little more.

If there's an upside to cancer, it's that most people will be empathetic, loving, and supportive when you are sick. Even your judgiest friends and harshest critics will rein it in and ease up on you. (The ones who don't are the ones you should reevaluate your friendship with.) I noticed this immediately. Coworkers, friends, family—they all stopped questioning me, got out of my way, and let me do what I wanted to do.

Rarely in our adult lives do we get this sort of freedom. When you are sick with cancer most people are willing to give you a reprieve, a "time-out," so to speak. This can be physical, mental, or if you're really lucky,

> *The question is: Now that you have a second chance at life—what are you going to do differently? How are you going to emerge from this cancer journey a stronger, smarter, more grateful person?*

both. My advice is, use this moment to your benefit. I used it as my "Get Out of Jail Free" card—an opportunity for a do-over at my life. I figured it was my second chance at life, so why waste it? I didn't like where my life was headed so I used this time to "press the brake and pivot." I quit my job, broke up with my long-term boyfriend, and started to approach life in a totally different way— one that helped me channel the best version of myself.

"That's the thing about cancer—everything sorta snaps into focus," says Hoda. "The BS falls by the wayside and you zero in on the top ten things that really mean something to you, things you really care about. They weren't the same as the day before your diagnosis. But if there is an upside to all this, it's that we get to reevaluate our lives, and that's a good thing."

Make no mistake—you define your life. The choices you make are *your* choices. Not making a choice is even a choice. The great news is—there are no wrong choices. Every choice you have made in the past, you made because it was the best choice for you at the time. This is a powerful, powerful fact. And it's a reason why you shouldn't have regrets in life. Oprah talks about this all the time on *Super Soul Sunday*.

Many of us—most, actually—don't know our own power. We come up with a million reasons why the choices are out of our control and how we are powerless to change our circumstances. But the fact is, you have power over most things in your life. You may not feel like you do, but you do.

The question is: Now that you have a second chance at life—what are you going to do differently? How are you going to emerge from this cancer journey a stronger, smarter, more grateful person?

"A lot of people don't have the luxury of today," says Sandra Lee, Emmy-winning lifestyle expert and DCIS breast cancer survivor. "Today might not be my best day. It might downright suck, but it's a day that I get and I don't take it for granted. Now, every single day, I ask myself, 'What did I do today worth giving my life for?' That's how I decide the work I am going to do, the friends I want around me and who I want to be."

I feel like my life is actually better after cancer. I say this all the time, "Cancer almost killed me but it really saved my life." Facing a major health crisis is life-altering because it gives you the opportunity to gain a different perspective. It made me reevaluate everything and I'm a happier person today because of it. Below are the eight rules I live by now that help me hold on to my happiness. They don't require money but they will make your life rich.

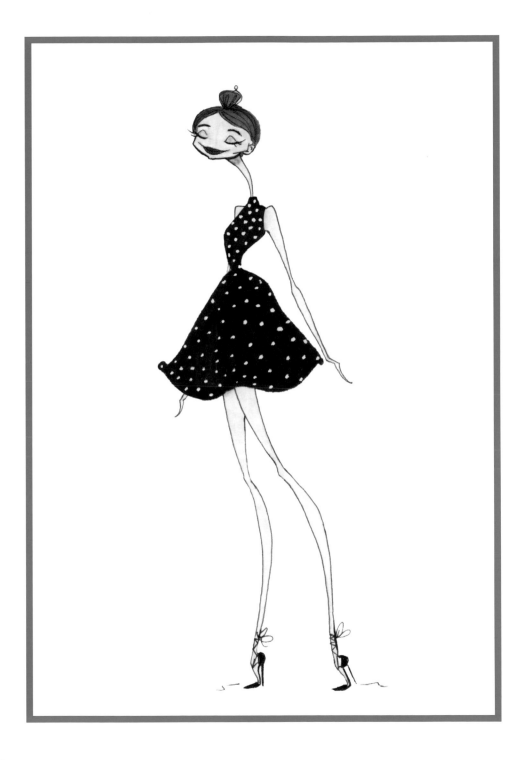

cait's great 8

1 express gratitude

Never let the things you want make you forget about the things you have. Your life is abundant once you really take a look at it. (If you are having trouble with this one, volunteer at a homeless shelter or a pediatric hospital floor. It won't take long to realize how blessed you really are.)

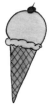

2 savor life's joys

The real beauty in life is in each precious moment. Stop and smell the roses. I advocate eating lots of chocolate croissants and enjoying long make-out sessions!

3 commit to goals

Most people who fail at reaching their dream, fail not from lack of ability but from lack of commitment. What's your passion project? Get it going! What are you waiting for?

4 cultivate optimism

When it rains, look for rainbows. When it's dark, look for stars. Both are beautiful. It's just perspective. Find the silver linings.

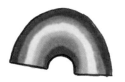

5 don't overthink things

Thinking too much complicates your life and creates a problem that wasn't even there in the first place. Quiet your mind.

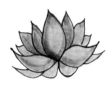

6 avoid social comparisons

Most of our insecurities and unhappiness come from comparing our behind-the-scenes with other people's highlight reel. Focus on making your journey meaningful. Ignore all that other crap. You are a unicorn after all!

7 increase flow experiences

Flow is a state where you are so focused it feels like time stands still. Doing what you love and challenging yourself are how you get there.

8 nurture your relationships

The happiest people alive have deep, meaning-ful relationships. Nurture them and watch them grow. It is never too late to do this. You can start right now…

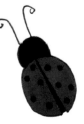

I want to end this chapter, this book, by urging you to use this moment as a time for personal growth and to find your happy. If you really do the work, I promise, you will emerge a better and more beautiful person for it. Remember, when you walk through hell you come out on fire.

> *It doesn't happen all at once," said the Skin Horse. "You become. It takes a long time. That's why it doesn't happen often to people who break easily, or have sharp edges, or who have to be carefully kept. Generally, by the time you are Real, most of your hair has been loved off, and your eyes drop out and you get loose in the joints and very shabby. But these things don't matter at all, because once you are Real you can't be ugly, except to people who don't understand.*

—THE VELVETEEN RABBIT BY MARGERY WILLIAMS

journal pages

ACKNOWLEDGMENTS

It often takes a game of telephone to connect you to the right people, who then in turn connect you to the right doctors. It is my telephone chain that I want to thank first: Luisa Marciano and Andrew Levy, Stacie Caplan-Kiratsous, Michelle Steinberg, Pam Kohl, and Myra Biblowit. Each of you (some who didn't even know me at the time) helped get me into the right medical hands with one act of compassion. Phone lines became lifelines and for this I am forever indebted to you.

To Dr. Eliza Port and Dr. Leo Keegan, my guardian angels on earth. It's rare to find doctors with your level of knowledge, expertise, and skill. Rarer yet, to find ones who are modest, compassionate, and will go above and beyond for their patients. I considered myself blessed to have been in your care. You gave me back my life—and with it—hope for a better future. I'm not even sure how to properly thank you for this. Hopefully, sharing your unparalleled advice is the way I can pay it forward.

To my fellow breast cancer "thrivers": Joan Lunden, Hoda Kotb, Sandra Lee, Suleika Jaouad, Elena Tavarez, Laura Rubin, Dayna Christison, Torva Durkin, and Elizabeth Myers. Thank you for lending your names and platforms to help me with this project and, ultimately, other cancer patients on this journey. Your strength, positivity, and ability to spread the love are inspiring. The world is a better place having you in it.

To my glam gang who was with me from the beginning of the journey: Ted Gibson, Ramy Gafni, Sonia Kashuk, Dr. Doris Day, Dr. Heidi Waldorf, Elle Gerstein, Dr. Brian Kantor, and Dr. Josh Zeichner. In many ways, I credit you for this book—because you reminded me that I had the right as a living, breathing human being to care about myself and my physical aesthetic while battling cancer. You empowered this ideology with knowledge, love, and product suggestions. You reminded me (often) that looking good isn't about vanity but about feeling better—emotionally and physically. This idea hasn't always been encouraged in the medical community, which makes your words more vital and reinforces why you are visionaries in the industry. I am a lucky girl to have you by my side—then and now.

To all the experts and institutions who took the time to be interviewed for this book, your contribution is impactful and appreciated: Dr. Richard Doty and the Smell and Taste Center at the Perelman School of Medicine at the University of Pennsylvania; Dr. Avery Gilbert and the University of Pennsylvania; Lisa Lewis and Givaudan; Dr. Mindy Greenstein and Memorial Sloan Kettering; Cutler Salon, Andrew DiSimone, and The Hair Place; Dr. Donald F. Richey and Brighter Days; Dr. Heidi Waldorf and Mount Sinai; Dr. Doris Day and NYU; Karen Hohenstein, Dr. Michele Halyard, and the Mayo Clinic/Mayo Medical School; Dr. Jeannette Graf; Dr. Brian Kantor and Lowenberg, Lituchy and Kantor; Dr. Ilene Bernstein and the University of Washington; Elle Gerstein; Dr. Dana Stern and Mount Sinai School of Medicine; Doug Schoon and Schoon Scientific; Dr. Jill Waibel and Baptist Hospital of Miami; Vinnie Myers; Wendy Williams; Daniele Hollywood; Dr. Jennifer Litton and University of Texas MD Anderson Cancer Center; Dr. Lauren F. Streicher and the Feinberg School of Medicine/Northwestern University/Northwestern Medicine Center for Sexual Medicine; Dr. Elizabeth Eden and the New York Gynecological Society; and Cindy Barshop.

To Tom " Mazz" Mazzarelli: You've been the same since high school—funny, sharp, and kind. Thank you, friend, for your never-ending generosity and support.

To Mark Weiss: Your iconic photographs of Ozzy, Debbie Harry, Eric Clapton, Journey, Boy George, Zappa, Kiss, U2—just to name a few—have had such a visual impact on my relationship with music and pop culture. Had anybody told me that I would one day get to sit for you—I wouldn't have believed it. But dreams do come true! Thank you for turning your lens on me and capturing this meaningful time in my life. It was a thrill I will never forget!

To Mike Levine, Terry Egan, and Dan Wakeford: You shaped my career as a journalist by teaching me how to channel my voice into written word, to tell stories and see the bigger picture—and most importantly—to learn my value in the process. This book is a direct result of your impact on my life. (Mike, wherever you are, I hope you are looking down beaming with pride.)

To Tara Parker-Pope: Thank you for taking the time to read a pitch sent in by random freelancer about the final phase of her cancer reconstruction. You saw the heart and guts of my story—long before it went viral—and gave me the opportunity to share my message. My NYT byline was the springboard for this book and I have only you to thanks for that.

To Kassie Bracken: We were strangers when you began chronicling my journey for the *New York Times* and today I am happy to call you my friend. I don't know anybody else who could make me show my tits to ten million people but that is the magic of your charm. Thank you for lending your talent to raising awareness about the final stages of reconstruction for cancer patients and for telling my story with such empathy, love, and visual genius.

To my amazing illustrator, Jamie Lee Reardon: From the first moment I saw your work, I hoped that one day I would be able to collaborate with you. Your talent is beyond breathtaking. Thank you for lending your vision, talent, and time to this project. I know your illustrations will make those who are sad and struggling, smile and feel a happy. This book wouldn't be the same without you—and I wouldn't want it any other way.

To my publishing team at Grand Central: They say it takes a village to make a book but a few talented and hardworking women are all you *really* need. Thank you to Jamie Raab, an early champion of this project, Deb Futter, Karen Murgolo, and Katherine Stopa. To the ladies who flipped through these pages countless times scrutinizing every little detail, I am beyond indebted: editor Brittany McInerney (OMG—what would I have done without you???), production editor Yasmin Mathew, and copy editor Justine Gardner. A big thanks to Daniella DeSanto, Nick Small, and Amanda Pritzker for all of your hard work spreading the love. To designer Danielle Young, for using your talent to bring this book to life—your work is truly spectacular. And a special thanks to my editor, Sarah Pelz: Your intuitive ability to offer advice with just the right amount of autonomy is something even this neophyte knows is both respectful and rare. I am proud and honored that you made me a part of the Hachette/Grand Central family. I hope we get to do this again soon.

To my agent, Lynn Johnston: You saw something in me, took a chance, and provided vital guidance throughout this intricate process. You are sharp, funny, and know your craft. You have been an inspiration to me both as a mentor and as a woman in business. I also know that I have only been able to achieve this dream of mine because you were in my corner. I am forever grateful.

To my publicist, Jennifer Fisherman Ruff: You were by my side during my darkest days when I was living this book. And here you still are! You are a class act in couture and I feel blessed having you in my life. Thank you for your unwavering love and support.

To my Girl Gang, Jesse "The Original JLo" LoBreglio, Carly Abel Ritter, Dana "D-Nice" Mendelowitz, Randi Friedman, Leah "Ginzy" Ginsberg, Juliette Levy, Nicole Martinez, Lara Eurdolian, Damian "Judy" Irizarry, and Victoria and Valentina Sanford. It's easy to call someone a friend but very few step up and do what it takes when shit gets real. You saw me through my worst and helped me be my best. I love you each of you so much.

To my family: The soldiers in the trenches with me. Your love and support mean everything. A special thanks to my sister, Moira Kiernan, who sat with me in chemo, held me in the shower when I was too weak to stand, brought me munchies, cozy pjs, and really depressing books (no doubt to make me think my life was not so terrible; smooth one, Mo) and when I was too high on meds to read, turned me onto the best bad TV. We may fight like cats and dogs but you are my blood and I will love you into our next lives. Until then, "Meet me in Montauk."

To my father, Paul, and Patty Kiernan: Watching the two of you handle Patty's cancer with fortitude, grace, and calm set the example for me during my own battle. I know I wasn't the easiest child but I hope I made you proud in the end. Thank you for your support.

To my mother, Deirdre "What Is Deirdre," and Bruce "Brudad" Birnbaum: Even when you were a single parent struggling to raise three girls, your devotion, love, and support never wavered. I truly believe that is the reason why we turned out to be smart, hardworking, and compassionate women. Thank you for always being there. (Pulling on my earlobe now.)

And lastly, to the love of my life, Kenny Kaplan: You changed the trajectory of my world with your love, patience, calming presence, thoughtful advice, encouragement, and support. And you have shared with me the greatest gifts—Carly and Jonah, who fill my life with such unimaginable joy. Thank you for being a wonderful father and partner.

REFERENCES

CHAPTER 1—this stinks! *how treatment affects your sense of smell*

Gilbert, Dr. Avery. *What the Nose Knows: The Science of Scent in Everyday Life.* New York: Crown, 2008.

Herz, Dr. Rachel. *The Scent of Desire: Discovering Our Enigmatic Sense of Smell.* New York: HarperCollins, 2007.

Hongratanaworakit, T. "Stimulating Effect of Aromatherapy Massage with Jasmine Oil." http://www.ncbi.nlm.nih.gov/pubmed/20184043. *US National Library of Medicine National Institutes of Health.* January 5, 2010.

CHAPTER 2—the mane event: *hair today, gone tomorrow*

Lunden, Joan. *Had I Known.* New York: HarperCollins, 2015.

CHAPTER 3—beauty is skin deep: *how to care for the skin you're in*

American Association for Cancer Research. "Botox Could Help Target Resistant Tumors for Treatment." *ScienceDaily.* February 15, 2006.

Day, Dr. Doris. *Forget the Facelift: Turn Back the Clock with Dr. Day's Revolutionary Four-Week Program for Ageless Skin.* New York: Penguin, 2005.

Graf, Dr. Jeannette. *Stop Aging, Start Living: The Revolutionary 2-Week pH Diet That Erases Wrinkles, Beautifies Skin, and Makes You Feel Fantastic.* New York: Harmony, 2008.

CHAPTER 4—getting mouthy: *let's chat about oral care*

Bernstein, I. L. "Learned Taste Aversions in Children Receiving Chemotherapy." *Science* 200, no. 4347 (June, 16, 1978).

CHAPTER 5—stay polished: *nail treatments you need to know about*

American Cancer Society. "Chemotherapy for Breast Cancer." Sept. 13, 2016, http://www.cancer.org/cancer/breastcancer/detailedguide/breast-cancer -treating-chemotherapy

Robert, Caroline, et al. "Nail Toxicities Induced by Systemic Anticancer Treatments." *The Lancet: Oncology* 16, no. 4 (April 2015).

Scotté, Florian, et al. "Multicenter Study of a Frozen Glove to Prevent Docetaxel-Induced Onycholysis and Cutaneous Toxicity of the Hand." *Journal of Clinical Oncology* 23, no. 19 (July 2005).

CHAPTER 6—tit talk: *surgery and reconstruction*

Kiernan, Caitlin. "A Tattoo That Completes a New Breast," *New York Times,* June 2, 2014.

Lunden, Joan. *Had I Known.* New York: HarperCollins, 2015.

Port, Dr. Eliza. *The New Generation Breast Cancer Book: How to Navigate Your Diagnosis and Treatment Options—and Remain Optimistic—in an Age of Information Overload.* New York: Random House, 2015.

https://www.ncbi.nlm.nih.gov/pmc/articles/PMC4182909/

Pusic, Andrew L., et al. "Measuring and Managing Patient Expectations for Breast Reconstruction: Impact on Quality of Life and Patient Satisfaction." *Expert Review of Pharmacoeconomics & Outcomes Research,* January 9, 2014, http://www.tandfonline.com/doi/full/10.1586/erp.11.105.

CHAPTER 7—makeup is the best medicine: *how color is curative*

Gafni, Ramy: *Ramy Gafni's Beauty Therapy: The Ultimate Guide to Looking and Feeling Great While Living with Cancer.* New York: M. Evans and Company, 2005.

CHAPTER 9—life after treatment

Streicher, Lauren F. *Sex Rx: Hormones, Health and Your Best Sex Ever and The Essential Guide to Hysterectomy.* New York: HarperCollins, 2015.

CHAPTER 10—happiness is a state of mind—relocate there!

Greenstein, Mindy. *The House on Crash Corner.* New York, Greenpoint Press, 2011.

Lee, I-Min, et al. "Effect of Physical Inactivity on Major Noncommunicable Diseases Worldwide: An Analysis of Burden of Disease and Life Expectancy." *The Lancet* 380, no. 9838 (July 18, 2012).

Shankar Mahadevan Academy. "Shlokas and Their Benefits," December 1, 2013, http://www.shankarmahadevanacademy.com/blog/Shlokas-and-their-Benefits/.

INDEX

ABOUT THE AUTHOR

Caitlin Kiernan is an award-winning journalist, beauty expert and cancer survivor. A former fashion columnist, "Fashion Plate Cait," at the *Times Herald-Record* (a Dow Jones newspaper), she has worked as a beauty director at *Life & Style Weekly* and beauty producer for *Style Code Live*. She has appeared on both national and local television programs and networks including *E! News*, *Access Hollywood*, *Entertainment Tonight*, *Fox News*, the Sundance Channel, *The Wendy Williams Show*, and Bravo's *Real Housewives of New York*. Her freelance work appears in *The Wall Street Journal*, *Women's Health*, *Men's Health*, *Fitness*, *Men's Journal*, *Maxim*, Refinery29, *SU2Cancer*, *StyleWatch*, *Dr. Oz The Good Life*, PBS, Yahoo! Travel, *Today*, *Harper's Bazaar*, and *The New York Times*. She lives in Riverdale, New York.